today to increase your
fertility

Foreword by Nim Barnes,
founder of Foresight

Sally Lewis

PERSONAL HEALTH GUIDES

50 THINGS YOU CAN DO TODAY TO INCREASE YOUR FERTILITY

Summersdale Publishers Ltd
46 West Street
Chichester
West Sussex
PO19 1RP
UK

www.summersdale.com

Printed and bound in Great Britain

ISBN: 978-1-84953-119-1

Substantial discounts on bulk quantities of Summersdale books are available to corporations, professional associations and other organisations. For details contact Summersdale Publishers by telephone: +44 (0) 1243 771107, fax: +44 (0) 1243 786300 or email: nicky@summersdale.com.

Disclaimer
Every effort has been made to ensure that the information in this book is accurate and current at the time of publication. The author and the publisher cannot accept responsibility for any misuse or misunderstanding of any information contained herein, or any loss, damage or injury, be it health, financial or otherwise, suffered by any individual or group acting upon or relying on information contained herein. None of the opinions or suggestions in this book are intended to replace medical opinion. If you have concerns about your health, please seek professional advice.

Other titles in the Personal Health Guides series include:

50 Things You Can Do Today to Manage Anxiety
50 Things You Can Do Today to Manage Arthritis
50 Things You Can Do Today to Manage Back Pain
50 Things You Can Do Today to Manage Eczema
50 Things You Can Do Today to Manage Hay Fever
50 Things You Can Do Today to Manage IBS
50 Things You Can Do Today to Manage Insomnia
50 Things You Can Do Today to Manage Migraines
50 Things You Can Do Today to Manage Menopause

Acknowledgements

I would like to thank everyone involved in this book, including Nim Barnes at Foresight for her expert advice and insight into the issues that can affect fertility. To Jennifer Barclay and her team at Summersdale, especially my editor Anna Martin for her support, encouragement and helpful suggestions that helped create this book. Thanks also to my agent Isabel Atherton, and the numerous clients and couples who told me their fertility secrets and problems. And finally I'd like to thank my family for their continued support.

Contents

1. Understand your fertility
2. Keep your hormones balanced
3. Recognise your fertile time
4. Get your timing right
5. Monitor your fertility
6. Check his fertility
7. Consider your biological clock
8. Learn about infertility
9. Visit your GP

10. Choose low-GI foods
11. Balance your hormones with B vitamins
12. Know your fats
13. Power up with protein
14. Increase your fibre intake
15. Drink water

Author's Note

For many years I have been teaching conception and birth classes to numerous women, both within and outside of the NHS. Many of them have spoken of wishing they had access to more information about understanding their fertility; for some, becoming pregnant was a frustrating and difficult journey, taking much longer than expected.

Indeed it took several attempts for me to conceive and get past the 12-week stage before I eventually gave birth to a son. Prior to trying to conceive again, I decided I should learn more about my own fertility; which lifestyle factors affected it, the importance of my diet and how I could maximise my chances of becoming pregnant. By the time I next conceived – another very healthy boy – I had changed my lifestyle and was taking herbal supplements and eating a balanced diet.

I wrote this fertility book to offer easily accessible information. It suggests the lifestyle changes you may need to adopt, the diet you may need to consider and the treatment and options you may have to contemplate to be able to successfully conceive. I wish you all good luck in your quest for a healthy baby.

Sally Lewis

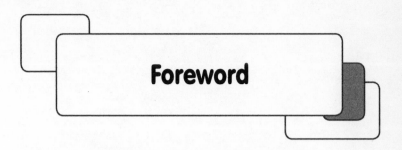

Foreword

By Nim Barnes, founder of Foresight

There is a great deal in this book that will be really useful to all couples hoping to have a baby, which is by far one of the most joyful and exciting experiences in life.

Yes, it is important to get everything right; the healthier the sperm and ova, the stronger the uterus and the better the outcome is likely to be.

At Foresight we have been looking after couples with fertility issues for the last 32 years. Some couples have spent many years pursuing their dream of starting a family, and they come to us mentally and physically exhausted.

Many of the ideas in Sally's book echo those of Foresight. This book is well worth reading; it is full of valuable advice for all couples hoping to conceive and I wish all readers the best of luck in starting or adding to their family.

Introduction

What is fertility?

Fertility is a woman's ability to become pregnant, and a man's ability to make a woman pregnant. Generally, most couples don't think too much about reproduction and their fertility until they decide they want a family. For many of those couples the ability to conceive – that is the fertilisation of a woman's egg with a man's sperm – poses no problems at all; for many couples regular unprotected intercourse is all that is required to make a baby. Yet conception is a complex and delicate process, which is affected by a range of factors including age, weight, smoking, lifestyle, stress and even prescribed medication.

According to the Human Fertilisation and Embryology Authority (HFEA), approximately a quarter of couples will experience a period of infertility lasting a year or more, and some will continue to experience problems for longer. At least one in six couples will consult an infertility specialist, and approximately one in 80 babies in the UK are born as a direct result of *in vitro* fertilisation (IVF).

What is infertility?

Infertility is defined as 'failing to get pregnant after two years of regular unprotected sex', according to the National Institute for Health and Clinical Excellence (NICE), who consider that fertility problems affect one in seven couples in the UK, although approximately 84 per cent of women will get pregnant within a year if they are not using contraception and having regular sexual intercourse.

Why does infertility occur?
Getting pregnant isn't always easy, but if it doesn't happen within a few months of trying it doesn't mean that you have a 'fertility problem'. In fact, it is much more likely that you are not making love at the right times; during a woman's monthly cycle there are only two to three days when pregnancy can occur, so it's easy to see how those days can be missed.

There is also a strong link between fertility and modern lifestyles: convenience foods offer little nutritional value; work-life balance affects stress levels and all too often leads to unhealthy habits like smoking or drinking too much alcohol and consuming too much sugary food and drink. It is no wonder that modern men and women have a decreased sex drive and hormonal imbalances.

This book explains how biological, social, psychological, genetic and lifestyle factors all affect fertility. It offers practical advice and a holistic approach to help improve your fertility. You'll discover how eating a balanced diet rich in nutrients will help to support the reproduction system and redress the balance of hormones, and about the importance of exercise. You'll learn about the tests you can take to check for ovulation sperm levels, or the levels of environmental toxins you may be exposed to, along with the conventional tests that your GP or fertility expert may use to see what, if any, fertility problems you may have. There is also a section on medical treatments and assisted conception: what you are entitled to and what to ask as you embark on this journey, and who to turn to should you need further support and help along the way.

You'll learn strategies for dealing with the stress and anxiety you may experience from trying for a baby and receive information about appropriate supplements and complementary therapy techniques that you might find beneficial. At the end of the book you will find details of useful organisations, helpful products, books and other sources of advice and support.

Pregnancy and age

A woman's ability to become pregnant decreases with age. According to an assessment on fertility problems conducted by the National Collaborating Centre for Women's and Children's Health, women are at their most fertile in their early 20s, when only approximately 7 per cent will have trouble conceiving. Between the ages of 35 and 39, 20 per cent of women are considered infertile and by the age of 40 this rises to 29 per cent.

Chapter 1

Fertility Matters

This chapter explains just what is meant by fertility, the menstrual cycle and ovulation, as well as the role of your reproductive hormones, your body's natural fertility signs and the best time for trying to conceive.

Understanding your monthly cycle and knowing exactly when you ovulate will increase your chances of conceiving, yet for many women this is not as easy as it seems.

According to the Human Fertilisation and Embryology Authority (HFEA), only 20 per cent of couples achieve pregnancy within the first month. In fact, it often takes numerous well-timed cycles before pregnancy is achieved and 10 per cent of women will not be pregnant after a year of trying.

1. Understand your fertility

Fertility is a natural, simple and yet complex series of events, which require a woman's egg and a man's sperm to make and produce a baby. A woman's fertility is based around her menstrual cycle, and although the average menstrual cycle is 28 days, this may not be the case for you. Knowing when you are most likely to be ovulating is one of the most important factors in determining when you are most fertile and likely to conceive. Given that there is a very limited period of time when you are actually fertile during your cycle, it is clear why understanding your menstrual cycle is so important. Some women may have a regular cycle of 20 days or less, others 21 or more, but as long as your cycle is regular and consistent, then ovulation and conception are much more likely. If your cycle is sporadic or fluctuates in length each month, you may find becoming pregnant is more difficult. If you have been on the pill for a considerable period of time, you may find it takes you longer to know what your regular menstrual cycle is; however, once you do, the likelihood is that you will improve your chances of conceiving.

Your menstrual cycle

The length of your menstrual cycle is measured from the first day of your period, which may be indicated by the first signs of spotting, to the day before your next period starts, and your fertility will vary depending on the length of your cycle. The time from ovulation to your next period is likely to be constant – usually 10–16 days – but the time before you ovulate can be variable. You can identify the fertile time in your cycle either by observing your cervical secretions or recording your temperature, or knowing the position of your cervix, which will be discussed in this chapter. Only if your cycle is a regular 28 days will you ovulate mid-cycle, around day 14; if your cycle is 25 days then ovulation is around day 11; and if your cycle is longer, ovulation will also be later. Very often, women mistake the middle of their cycle and miss the most fertile time for conception to occur.

Your eggs

Your eggs are created when you yourself are in the womb, and a woman's supply of eggs – initially several millions – is depleted by the time of puberty. During your fertile life approximately 400 eggs will be released through ovulation, and by the time of your menopause your egg supply will have been used up. The eggs are kept within your ovaries and, every month, several eggs develop although usually only one develops to maturity; the rest simply degenerate. The mature egg, also known as the ovum, is released from one ovary, and is ready for fertilisation within the next 12–24 hours. If the egg is successfully fertilised, it then has to implant itself into the wall of the uterus, which results in pregnancy.

Ovulation

Simply put, ovulation is the release of one or maybe two eggs (ova) from the ovarian follicle and is the most likely time in your menstrual cycle for you to become pregnant. Although approximately 15 eggs may mature inside the ovaries each month, generally only the largest is released from a follicle in the ovary and travels down the Fallopian tube. Ovulation does not follow a regular pattern between both ovaries every month: which ovary releases the egg is relatively arbitrary. Once released, the egg has to be fertilised within 12–24 hours before it begins to degenerate. The egg develops in a fluid-filled sac called the follicle following stimulation from oestradiol, the primary form of oestrogen.

If your cycle is regular, you will be able to work out when you are ovulating and you can certainly use an ovulation calendar or an ovulation predictor kit to help you out. However, there are also a number of physical changes that occur in your body during ovulation and these can be used to help identify when you are ovulating so that you can time intercourse accordingly. They include:

- Changes in your cervical mucus, which will be explained later in this chapter
- Breast tenderness

- Bloating
- Increased sex drive
- A rise in body temperature
- Mild abdominal pain

The role of your hormones

Your menstrual cycle is governed by your pituitary gland. Located in the brain, this important master gland secretes hormones (chemicals) that travel through your body in your bloodstream and control your temperature, growth, thyroid activity, urine and production of testosterone (in men), oestrogen and progesterone (in women). It is these hormones, which stimulate the ovaries, the adrenal glands and men's testes that play an important role in your fertility.

Phases of your menstrual cycle

Your cycle is split into two distinct phases, the follicular phase and the luteal phase.

Follicular phase

On day one of your cycle, the first day of your period, the brain releases gonadotrophin, which in turn stimulates the pituitary gland to release follicle-stimulating hormone (FSH). This hormone does exactly as its name implies: it stimulates the immature eggs within the follicles to start growing.

The levels of FSH build up over the next couple of weeks. As the eggs grow and mature, they secrete oestrogen, one of the main female hormones that control the reproductive system, which stimulates the lining of the uterus, the endometrium, to thicken, preparing it for the onset of pregnancy. The oestrogen levels continue to rise as the eggs mature and FSH production decreases, ensuring only one egg continues to develop; the other eggs simply fade and die and, as you approach the middle of your cycle, a surge of lutenising hormone (LH) from the pituitary gland is released. This LH surge stimulates ovulation, causing the follicle to rupture, releasing the egg onto the surface of the ovary. Once the LH peaks, the corpus luteum begins to pump progesterone out, causing your body to heat up: your temperature rises as your body prepares a warm, welcoming environment for your baby. At the same time, your cervix is high, soft and open and changes occur in your cervical mucus so the sperm are able to pass through the cervix to reach the ovum.

Luteal phase

Once the follicular phase is over, the reproductive hormone progesterone is produced by the corpus luteum, a part of the ovary from which the mature egg bursts during ovulation. The production of progesterone prevents LH and FSH production and continues to thicken the endometrium in preparation for a fertilised egg, developing the structures that provide nutrients to the embryo.

A fertilised egg will stay in your Fallopian tube for between six to eight days after conception and the developing embryo grows as it travels down the Fallopian tube. It is known as a blastocyst by the time it implants itself in the womb lining. Sometimes this can cause minor bleeding or spotting. Changes within the womb include the development of special protrusions known as chorionic villi. These villi produce the hormone human chorionic gonadotrophin (hCG), which increases the size of the corpus luteum and produces more progesterone, thus maintaining the pregnancy. It is hCG that pregnancy tests detect to determine if you are pregnant.

If pregnancy does not occur, then both oestradiol and progesterone production decline approximately seven days after ovulation, resulting in menstrual bleeding as the endometrium is shed, approximately two weeks after ovulation, and the cycle starts all over again.

Hormones

Hormones are chemical messengers that are carried in the bloodstream and trigger activity in different organs of the body. The reproductive hormones control your monthly cycle and help to maintain pregnancy.

2. Keep your hormones balanced

Your reproductive hormones, namely oestrogen and progesterone for women and testosterone for men, play a very important role in fertility but can be easily affected by stress, lifestyle, lack of sleep, poor diet and other environmental factors, such as chemicals and toxins in food packaging and cosmetics. If these hormones become imbalanced, fertility can be adversely affected, lowering your chances of conceiving or staying pregnant once conception has occurred. It is helpful to try to recognise hormonal fluctuations during your cycle to increase your awareness of your fertility. Chapter 2 looks at foods that can help and Chapter 3 offers some practical solutions for dealing with some of these problems.

3. Recognise your fertile time

Your body will give you some clear signals when it is more fertile than at other times. Trying to interpret these signals can sometimes prove challenging so it is always worthwhile seeking medical advice. A fertility awareness nurse at a family planning clinic can help you to understand your monthly cycle, but there are several other factors, listed below, which may be used independently or in conjunction with each other. If you find you have difficulty interpreting them, ask a fertility nurse for advice.

Record your menstrual cycle

Keep a chart, record or diary of your menstrual cycle for several months before trying for a baby if you can, as this will help you identify ovulation. You can also write down your feelings during each month, looking for hormonal swings and mood changes that may indicate an imbalance in your hormones.

Use an ovulation calendar

Predicting your ovulation period can enhance your chances of becoming pregnant. The easiest and simplest method is to simply count the days leading to ovulation. It helps if you have a regular cycle, but also if you understand your cycle. You can use an online ovulation calendar, such as www.babyhopes.com/ovulation-calendar. html or www.ovulation-calendar.net, which will work it out for you.

Take your temperature

Your temperature rises in the middle of your cycle, confirming that ovulation has taken place. Taking your temperature can prove helpful for many women trying to identify their most fertile period and the easiest type of thermometer to use is an electronic digital thermometer, available from pharmacists.

Take your temperature first thing in the morning, before you get out of bed: this is your basal body temperature; your temperature naturally rises during the day. By taking your temperature at around the same time every day, you may be able to identify a rise resulting from ovulation. Just after ovulation there should be a rise of approximately 0.4–0.6°F (0.2°C). It may be necessary for you to chart several cycles so that you can see an emerging pattern. If your cycle is regular and based on 28 days, you should have a temperature rise around days 14–16, due to increased levels of progesterone; however, you will be most fertile just before this rise. Count the days from your last period and aim for intercourse every other day between days 11 and 16.

Several other factors can affect your temperature, particularly illness, alcohol, high stress levels, doing shift work, taking drugs and lack of sleep. These should be borne in mind if you decide to use temperature as a way of charting your cycle.

Basal body temperature

The average body temperature is 37°C (98.6°F), but anything from 36.5°C (97.7°F) to 37.2°C (99°F) is considered normal. A high temperature of 38°C (100°F) or above is considered likely to be a fever and should be measured again after two to three hours to see if you should seek medical attention.

Cervical secretions

Most fertility experts agree that your cervical secretions are the most accurate indicators of your most fertile time and Jane Knight, a fertility nurse specialist at the Zita West Clinic in London (see Directory), runs classes to teach women how to interpret the changes that take place in mucus secretions. According to research, the presence of cervical secretions is linked to a twofold increase in the probability of conception. For some women this self-inspection can be a little daunting and obviously to self-examine you must have clean hands and fingers, as you test the elasticity of the mucus between your thumb and forefinger (the fingertip test).

The mucus-secreting glands lining your cervical canal produce mucus continually, but these secretions alter as you approach ovulation. It is likely you will notice them as your vagina becomes more slippery and wet as ovulation approaches, although they can vary from one cycle to another, so it is worthwhile charting or recording them over a few cycles to be able to recognise the changes. There will be an increase in mucus which will become clear, stretchy or elastic, and will resemble egg white. This is fertile mucus and provides the ideal conditions for the sperm to reach its destination and fertilise an egg. Sperm can live in this mucus for up to seven days as it is much more alkaline at this time, protecting the sperm from the normal acidity of the vagina. Once ovulation is over, the secretions revert back to a thicker, creamier secretion that forms a seal over the cervix to prevent sperm or bacteria from entering.

If you cannot find any fertile mucus, you may be ovulating early; ovulation is affected by oestrogen levels, and low oestrogen levels, common in women during the lead up to the menopause, can begin any time during your mid-30s, but can also occur if your diet is too high in wheat fibre or if your body weight is too low. Other factors that can cause low oestrogen levels include too much exercise, smoking, taking antibiotics, a vitamin A deficiency and taking the contraceptive pill over a period of several years.

However, you can improve your mucus secretions by eating foods high in vitamin B (see Chapter 2) and drinking plenty of water.

Lower abdominal discomfort

It is thought that approximately one fifth (20 per cent) of fertile women actually feel ovulatory activity, which can range from mild aches to sharp pain on one side only. This ovulation symptom may last from a few minutes to a few hours.

Cervix changes

Oestrogen and progesterone cause changes in your cervix, which you can learn to recognise by feeling your cervix with your fingers at the same time each day. When your fertility is at its highest your cervix will feel high, soft and open, as opposed to low, hard and closed at other times of the month. A fertility nurse at your local family planning clinic should be able to help you with this.

4. Get your timing right

It's not just a case of having sex when your fertility is at its peak; you can have sex as often as you like throughout your cycle, but if you are finding that your lovemaking is not hitting the right spot then you may find that your chances of getting pregnant will increase if you have unprotected sex during your peak fertility time; the ovulation period of your cycle. Aim to have sex, and lots of it, three to four days before ovulation, so that the sperm are ready and waiting. They can live in your body for this period and your egg can live for up to 40 hours after being released. Your most fertile period usually starts four to five days before ovulation and ends approximately 24–48 hours after ovulation.

How often should we try?

Guidance from NICE suggests you should have sex every two to three days throughout the month if you are trying to conceive.

5. Monitor your fertility

There are a number of products on the market these days to help you monitor your fertility, enabling you to plan ahead and schedule the right time for intercourse. They include the new DuoFertility monitor, a temperature sensor the size of a £1 coin, worn as a patch under the arm, that downloads data to a hand-held reader, revealing your fertility for the forthcoming week. The data is then downloaded to the company, where a fertility expert will analyse it for you. According to the company which makes the monitor, the device is so sensitive that it can be used to forecast fertile days for women with irregular cycles and could be useful for those suffering from polycystic ovary syndrome (PCOS). DuoFertility is available from www.duofertility. com. Other fertility monitors can be found at Boots (www.boots. com), and www.fertilityfriend.com offers support and advice.

Ovulation predictor kits

There are several types of do-it-yourself ovulation kits on the market to help you identify the most fertile period within your cycle. While there is no evidence that they will naturally improve your chances of success in becoming pregnant, they may help predict your ovulation, especially if your cycle is irregular. There are two types of these kits: one tests your urine and the other your saliva. They are available over the counter without the need for a prescription. They can also be bought online at www.clearblue.com or www.firstresponsefertility.com.

Urine hormone tests

This test will help identify the increase or surge of LH levels that occur a day or two before ovulation. Although there is always a trace of LH in your urine and blood, this will increase between two to five times before ovulation. The 12–36-hour period between the beginning of the LH surge and your egg being released is the most fertile part of your cycle and the time when you are most likely to conceive. Research shows that urine hormone kits can accurately predict ovulation; however, if you have low or high levels of LH, they may not be so reliable.

Urine kits include the Clearblue Digital Ovulation Test (www. clearblue.com) and the Babystart FertilTime Ovulation Kit, available from www.babystart-eco.co.uk.

Saliva-based ovulation predictor kits

These kits test for rising oestrogen levels and increased salt in your saliva as you get closer to ovulation. They are pocket-sized microscopes, which you use to see if 'salivary ferning' (a fern-like pattern of salt in your saliva as you near ovulation) has occurred. They are not as reliable as the urine ovulation predictor kits. Saliva tests are available from www.babystart.co.uk and www.homehealth-uk.com.

6. Check his fertility

Unlike women, men can be fertile all the time. From puberty, they manufacture sperm constantly; an adult man produces millions of sperm every day and, just like women, men produce both FSH and LH hormones but, unlike women, they do so at a constant rate throughout the month. A man's fertility depends on the balance between FSH and LH being maintained at all times. Testosterone is a hormone required by men for sexual function.

Improving sperm quality

Although you may not know at this stage whether your man is fertile or not, simple lifestyle changes can significantly improve the quality of his sperm. Sperm are adversely affected by alcohol, excess weight, diet, sexually transmitted diseases, prescription medication, drugs, smoking, heat, environmental toxins and stress.

Sperm take approximately 100 days to develop, 74 days to form and 20–30 days to mature. Ideally, he should try to improve his sperm for 100 days before you start trying to conceive.

Good, healthy sperm require three essential factors:

1. A high count (anything above 20 million sperm per millilitre of ejaculation is good).

2. Good motility (the speed at which the sperm swim forward).

3. A healthy shape.

Anything that helps to reduce the adverse effects mentioned above will have a beneficial outcome on your partner's sperm. For example, reducing his alcohol and caffeine intake and stopping smoking will make a real difference, as will making sure he does not have long hot baths or spend long periods in saunas or jacuzzis, as this will damage sperm. It is thought that 40 per cent of sperm damage is caused by free-oxidising radicals; vitamins A, C and E, beta-carotene, selenium and zinc are known to protect sperm from this type of damage. (See Chapter 2 for more information).

Sperm production can also be affected by damage to the testicles, an obstruction such as a hernia, an infection or disease, sterilisation, hormone problems, ejaculation problems, mumps or hypogonadism – where there is an abnormally low production of testosterone.

Spermatozoa

Healthy sperm can live for up to seven days in the female reproductive tract. But your egg will only survive for about 12–24 hours if it is not fertilised. Fertilisation is possible for up to three days before ovulation. Even if a man ejaculates up to 300 million sperm at a time, only about two hundred of them will reach a Fallopian tube and have the chance to fertilise an egg.

7. Consider your biological clock

Although a man's age may have some impact on his fertility, a woman's age is much more significant when trying to conceive. Your age affects your fertility, which will begin to decline during your mid-30s. According to NHS statistics, 95 per cent of women who are

35 years old will get pregnant after three years of having regular unprotected sex, while only 75 per cent of women aged 38 will conceive after having regular unprotected sex over the same period.

As you age, the chance of getting pregnant with each cycle varies; medically, this is known as 'fecundability' – the ability to conceive. Statistics produced by the HFEA show that if you are aged between 20 and 25, your chance of getting pregnant per cycle is about 25 per cent; between 25 and 30 your chances are about 20 per cent; and between 30 and 35 they are 15 per cent. However, fecundability declines rapidly from 35 and your chance of pregnancy may reduce to 10 per cent per cycle, with a further decline the older you get. Based on these statistics, a woman under 30 will get pregnant within six cycles; by her early 30s it usually takes about nine cycles; and if she is in her mid-30s it will take approximately a year.

8. Learn about infertility

Infertility is when a couple cannot conceive despite having regular unprotected sex. According to the HFEA, around one in seven couples in the UK may have difficulty conceiving. However, the number of couples who are actually infertile is relatively low: approximately 5 per cent. Statistics show that about 85 per cent of couples will conceive naturally within one year if they have regular unprotected sex and 95 per cent will conceive within two years.

A couple will only be diagnosed as being infertile if they have not managed to conceive after two years of trying. There are two types of infertility:

Primary infertility: where someone who has never conceived a child in the past has difficulty conceiving.

Secondary infertility: where a person has had one or more babies in the past, but is having difficulty conceiving again.

For more information on infertility and medical treatment, see Chapter 6.

9. Visit your GP

If you are under 35 and have been having unprotected regular sex every two to three days throughout your cycle for the last year and have still not conceived, then it is worth booking an appointment to see your GP, who will arrange a series of tests for both of you. However, women who are over 35 and have been having unprotected sex for the last six months and have still not conceived should book an appointment with their GP as it becomes more difficult to become pregnant the older you get.

Chapter 2

Eat a Fertility-boosting Diet

It is now widely accepted that there is a direct link between the foods we eat and our physical and mental health, but little emphasis is placed on the importance of the food we need to make a baby. In the UK, some £500 million is spent on medical procedures to assist conception, yet little in terms of medical advice is offered to couples to understand the necessary nutrients their bodies require to conceive. Many couples may embark on assisted conception techniques not realising their diet and lifestyle factors may be preventing both ovulation and sperm production. Research undertaken by the University of Surrey in 1995 on behalf of Foresight, the Association for the Promotion of Preconceptual Care, looked at the progress of 367 couples trying to conceive. The women in the study were aged between 22 and 45 and the men from 25 to 59. Thirty-seven per cent of the couples had a history of infertility. All couples followed a healthy diet, which included eliminating smoking and alcohol and following an individually tailored vitamin and mineral supplementation programme. By the end of the three-year trial, 327 couples (89 per cent) had given birth, and 81 per cent of those with a history of infertility had conceived. A further study undertaken by a private fertility clinic had a success rate for assisted conception of 50 per cent when patients received both conventional and complementary medicine, which included a nutritional programme and tailored vitamin and mineral supplementation. The average national success rate for assisted conception is approximately 15 per cent.

Eating a healthy, balanced, nutritious diet enables your body to function effectively; the female menstrual cycle is directly influenced by your nutritional status, as is the production of healthy sperm. Women who eat too little and are underweight will often have irregularities with menstruation, problems with ovulation and in some cases no periods at all (amenorrhoea). Those who are considered overweight or have a body mass index (BMI) of 25 and above are likely to have raised oestrogen levels, which prevent ovulation. Fertility experts all agree that by reducing caffeine and avoiding additives and preservatives, such as artificial sweeteners, which upset blood sugar levels and disrupt hormonal balance, you can improve your fertility.

This chapter looks at how eating a balanced, nutritious diet can help influence hormonal balance and production. It also outlines the vitamins, minerals, fats and essential fatty acids you need for a healthy reproductive system, including B vitamins, antioxidant vitamins A, C and E, vitamin D, zinc, selenium, folic acid, magnesium and amino acids, and the foods you will find them in. The role of protein and carbohydrates are also discussed, along with the foods required to regulate blood sugar levels, helping you to deal with stress and reduce anxiety. The importance of fibre and water are also considered in this chapter.

10. Choose low-GI foods

We hear a lot about a balanced diet these days, but understanding just what that is can be confusing. Eating a low glycaemic index (GI) diet will help to maintain steady glucose levels and help prevent fluctuations in blood sugar levels, which can affect your mood, leaving you anxious and emotional. The GI is a measure of how quickly a food raises the level of sugar in the blood. Foods with a lower GI have widespread beneficial effects on general health, reducing the risk of heart disease and diabetes and lowering high cholesterol levels. High-GI foods, such as white bread, pasta and rice, increase blood sugar levels rapidly, and then they plummet. Low-GI foods, such as wholemeal bread, meat, cheese, eggs and pulses, keep blood sugar levels lower and more stable for a longer period.

A low-GI diet is considered to be beneficial for women suffering from PCOS, which directly affects fertility. Chapter 5 offers more information on PCOS.

11. Balance your hormones with B vitamins

There are several B vitamins that are vital for fertility as they help to regulate hormones and produce the body's genetic material (DNA and RNA). Deoxyribonucleic acid (DNA) is the genetic, hereditary material of a cell. Chromosomes inside a cell are made of DNA and are divided into sections. These sections are genes, which carry the instructions for making up the human body. RNA is ribonucleic acid and is very similar to DNA but is more involved in protein synthesis. Unfortunately, many lifestyle factors such as alcohol, stress, smoking and antibiotics can inhibit the absorption of these important vitamins, so supplementation can be very worthwhile. See Chapter 3 for more information on taking supplements.

The main B vitamins worth supplementing include B1, B2, B5, B6 and B12.

B1 (thiamine) – this is found in whole grains, nuts, brown rice, egg yolks, fish, poultry, pulses and seeds. A deficiency in this vitamin has been linked to failed ovulation.

B2 (riboflavin) – this is used by the liver to clear away used-up hormones, including oestrogen and progesterone. Without sufficient levels of B2, the levels of these hormones may fall, which may affect your fertility. Good food sources are similar to those for vitamin B1.

B5 (pantothenic acid) – this is vital around the time of conception and for foetal development. Good food sources include wheatgerm, salmon, broccoli, sweet potato, oranges, strawberries and nuts.

B6 (pyridoxine) – along with zinc, vitamin B6 is essential for the formation and functioning of oestrogen and progesterone. When there is a deficiency of B6, the ovaries will slow down the production of progesterone. Studies have shown that if women who have problems conceiving take a B6 supplement for a six-month period, their fertility can improve. Good food sources include whole grains, nuts, brown rice, egg yolks, fish, poultry, pulses and seeds and leafy green vegetables.

B12 – this is necessary, along with vitamin B9 (folic acid or folate), for the synthesis of DNA and the metabolism of cells. B12 maximises the uptake of folic acid, which is advised by the Department of Health as a supplement to be taken if you are trying to conceive. It is found only in animal products, including lamb, liver, poultry, salmon and sardines. Vegetarians may get this vitamin if their dairy intake is high, but many may require supplementation. B12 has also been shown to help improve a low sperm count.

Folic acid

Folic acid is water-soluble vitamin B9 and is used to fortify some foods, such as breakfast cereals and bread. Folic acid is also known as folate, when it occurs naturally in foods like cooked black-eyed beans and pulses, leafy green vegetables, granary bread, lettuce, oranges and tomatoes.

The Department of Health recommends that if you are trying for a baby you need more folic acid than you can get from your diet naturally. A 0.4 mg daily supplement of folic acid is recommended until the end of the twelfth week of pregnancy. Folic acid helps to prevent neural tube defects such as spina bifida, where the baby's spine does not form properly. However, research has shown that folic acid is just as important for men as for women, because it is required for healthy sperm, a good sperm count and motility. It is worth noting that folic acid is available on prescription.

PABA

Para-aminobenzoic acid (PABA) is a B-complex component that is thought to be of benefit for folate production. Research has long linked PABA to male fertility and it can be found in liver, whole grains, spinach, brewer's yeast and mushrooms.

Avoid soy products

It is thought that soy products may have mild contraceptive properties. They are not recommended if you are trying to get pregnant.

12. Know your fats

Fat produces hormones and aids the absorption and transportation of fat-soluble nutrients and vitamins around the body. According to research, fats are required for ovulation, so you need to eat sufficient fat for your body to function efficiently. However, it's important to eat the right type of fat in the right proportion.

There are four types of fat found in the foods we eat: trans, saturated, polyunsaturated (omega-3 and omega-6) and monounsaturated (omega-9).

1. Trans fats are the most damaging type of fat, and can be found in most margarines and in processed foods like biscuits, cakes and pastries. They are partially hydrogenated fats, which are formed when liquid vegetable oil is turned into solid fat through a process known as hydrogenation. These fats are thought to adversely affect ovulation and may make it more difficult to become pregnant.

2. Saturated fats are solid at room temperature and are thought to raise the levels of harmful low-density lipoprotein (LDL) cholesterol, which very often leads to hardening of the arteries and cardiovascular disease, obesity and an increased risk of some cancers. They can be found in foods such as red meat, and full-fat dairy products, including butter, cream, milk and ice cream.

3. Polyunsaturated fats can be divided into two types, omega-3 fatty acid and omega-6 fatty acid, and are also known as essential fatty acids (EFAs). They are beneficial for increasing fertility as they make prostaglandins, beneficial hormone-like regulating substances, increase cervical secretions, promote ovulation and improve the overall quality of the uterus by increasing blood flow to the reproductive organs. Omega-3 also helps to improve blood flow to the genitals and is vital for reproduction, while omega-6 can assist fertility by improving reproductive cell structure, reduces inflammation and helps to maintain the reproductive system. These fats can be found in fish, wholegrain wheat, margarine, peanut butter and sunflower seeds.

4. Monounsaturated fats lower low-density lipoprotein and raise high-density lipoprotein (HDL) levels. They are primarily found in plant oils such as olives, canola oils, avocados, peanuts and most other nuts, which are beneficial but high in calories.

Essential fatty acids

The fats and oils we eat are broken down into fatty acids, but essential fatty acids (EFAs) are fatty acids that we have to eat as the body cannot manufacture them. They are needed for cell structure and the production of cell membranes in the ovaries. Omega-3 EFAs have a derivative called docosahexaenoic acid (DHA), which most women are deficient in. Along with omega-6, DHA helps to form body tissues and is an important structural element of cell membranes.

Good food sources of omega-3 include oily fish like salmon, mackerel, trout, pilchards and sardines which can be canned or fresh. Fresh tuna is also an oily fish; however, when canned its fatty acids are reduced and it no longer counts as an oily fish. Other good food sources of omega-3 include canola oils, flax oil or spreads made from these oils, leafy green vegetables, hummus and eggs.

Good food sources of omega-6 include nuts, especially walnuts and Brazil nuts, and seeds, including sunflower and sesame seeds. They are also found in borage oil, corn oil, sunflower oil and safflower oil.

Best sources therefore include fish, especially oily fish, flaxseed oil, nuts and seeds. But do bear in mind that cooking can destroy EFAs.

Docosahexaenoic acid
Docosahexaenoic acid (DHA) is an omega-3 fatty acid found naturally only in oily fish, such as sardines, salmon, herring, mackerel, pilchard

and fresh (not tinned) tuna. It is known to have a significant effect on the health of sperm membranes. Research shows that infertile men have a much lower level of DHA in their sperm cells compared to fertile men, resulting in low motility and misshapen sperm.

Getting the balance right

Achieving the right balance between the two essential fatty acids is important; too much omega-6 can interfere with the body's ability to break down omega-3. As most cooking oils and margarines contain corn oil and sunflower oil, most British diets tend to be higher in omega-6. Try using olive oil and olive oil-based margarines and spreads instead.

13. Power up with protein

Proteins are the building blocks of the body: they repair and renew cells, including eggs and sperm, transport nutrients around the body, make antibodies, produce hormones, encourage the growth of new tissue and repair body tissue. They are made of amino acids and are needed for good-quality egg production and for FSH and LH production. If you eat too little protein, the gonadotrophin-releasing hormone responsible for the release of both FSH and LH will be compromised and you may experience menstrual problems, particularly infrequent periods. Both men and women need approximately 60–70 g (2.2–2.5 oz) of protein a day; it should make up approximately 20 per cent of your daily diet.

Protein can be found in animal products, meat, fish, eggs and dairy and also in vegetables, lentils, beans, peas, seeds, nuts and brown rice. It is best to include protein in more than one meal during the day as it is released slowly into your bloodstream.

L-arginine

This amino acid helps to boost male fertility and is essential for sperm production and quality.

L-carnitine

This is another amino acid that is also essential for normal sperm function. According to research, the higher the levels of L-carnitine, the better the quality of the sperm.

Vegetarian option

Vegetarians can get sufficient protein in their diet by eating nuts, especially Brazil nuts, almonds and cashews, as well as pulses such as chickpeas (for example in hummus), lentils and beans, eggs (preferably organic), and fruit and vegetables.

14. Increase your fibre intake

It is not just cereals that provide you with fibre: a daily minimum of five portions of fresh fruit and vegetables should provide you with adequate amounts of fibre. Ideally, your daily intake should be 18 g (0.6 oz), although most people only manage about 12 g (0.4 oz) a day.

Fibre has great health benefits, including fewer bowel problems and a reduced risk of some cancers, diabetes, and heart disease. The fibre in whole grains, fruit and vegetables reduces excess oestrogen levels and clears old hormones and waste products from your body, preventing the build-up of toxins, chemicals and pesticides, which can affect fertility in both men and women. The best sources of fibre can be found in grains, fruits, vegetables, nuts, seeds and pulses; however, excess wheat fibre (bran) can rob the body of oestrogen and block the absorption of vital nutrients such as zinc, calcium and magnesium, all vital for fertility, so you should not eat too much of this.

15. Drink water

Water is so important to the body: it's actually the most important nutrient after oxygen. It makes up 70 per cent of your body and is needed for many different functions, including the production of energy, elimination of toxins, transportation of hormones and development of sperm and cervical mucus. You lose water from your body on a daily basis through sweat, urine and breathing, and dehydration over a period of time will direct water away from the ovaries and testes towards the essential organs, like the heart and brain. Experts recommend 1.5–2.5 litres of water daily, which can seem a lot, but fruit and vegetables contain water and can contribute to your daily intake. Herbal teas, juiced raw fruit and vegetables juices all count. Ideally, drink filtered or glass-bottled water, as tap water is chlorinated and contains chemicals, and water from plastic bottles may also contain chemicals that leach from the plastic.

16. Mind your minerals

Minerals are essential nutrients that your body needs to function efficiently. The most important minerals needed for fertility in both men and women are listed below.

Zinc

Zinc is an essential component of genetic material and a deficiency in it can reduce fertility. Zinc helps the female reproductive hormones, oestrogen and progesterone, to work more efficiently, and helps maintain a healthy menstrual cycle. For men, zinc is vital for maintaining the production of testosterone and a good sperm count and motility. A deficiency in zinc will decrease sperm production in men. Zinc can be found in shellfish, meat, whole grains and wheatgerm, sunflower seeds and oats. Vitamins B6 and C may aid the absorption of zinc but too much fibre, tea, coffee and alcohol can inhibit the take-up.

Iron

Low levels of iron are known to adversely affect ovulation and are a common cause of anaemia, which directly affects the menstrual cycle. Iron deficiency is known to be the most common of nutritional deficiencies; the daily recommended amount is 10–15 mg per day, but it is estimated that over 50 per cent of women worldwide get less than this amount. Good food sources of iron include red meat, poultry, eggs, fish, cherries, dried fruits, bread, broccoli and green leafy vegetables.

> ### Iron supplements
>
> Iron supplements can cause constipation. You may require an iron supplement if your levels are very low. However, the best method of increasing your iron levels is to eat a diet rich in iron.

Magnesium

Low levels of this mineral are associated with female infertility. Good food sources include bananas, green leafy vegetables, nuts and seeds. Magnesium is lost through eating processed foods such as white bread.

Selenium

This trace mineral is also an antioxidant and protects your body from free radicals. It is very important for male fertility as it is necessary for sperm formation and can increase sperm count. Good food sources include fresh tuna, herring, red meat, wheatgerm, whole grains, bran and walnuts.

17. Increase your vitamin intake

Eating plenty of fruit and vegetables will ensure your diet is high in antioxidants, especially vitamins A, C, D and E. Antioxidants are known to neutralise the damaging effects of free radicals and pollutants on brain and body cells. Fruit and vegetables also contain other nutrients such as B vitamins and necessary minerals; eating a variety of coloured fruit and vegetables helps to ensure you receive a wide range of nutrients and antioxidants.

Vitamin C

This is an antioxidant and helps prevent damage by free radicals to the body's cells. It has been found to be very important in enhancing sperm quality and protecting the sperm from damage. It is also thought to help women with a luteal phase defect (the second half of the menstrual cycle). A lack of this vitamin can also cause the sperm to clump together, making them less motile. Dr Marilyn Glenville, a leading women's health nutrition specialist, believes women taking the fertility drug Clomiphene, which helps to stimulate ovulation, have a better chance of ovulating if they take vitamin C at the same time. Good food sources include oranges, strawberries, tomatoes and broccoli.

Vitamin E

Vitamin E is an antioxidant that benefits both men's and women's fertility by making sperm more fertile and improving ovulation.

Good food sources of vitamin E include cold-pressed oils, wheatgerm, whole grains, meat, eggs, sweet potatoes, leafy green vegetables, nuts, seeds and avocados. If you take a vitamin E supplement, look for the natural type (d-alpha-tocopherol), as this is more easily used and retained by the body. Zita West, a renowned fertility expert and midwife, suggests taking vitamin E with selenium and vitamin C to promote a healthy endometrium (the mucus membrane lining the womb).

Vitamin D

Research has shown a link between low levels of vitamin D and problems with ovulation. Vitamin D is produced in the skin after exposure to natural sunlight; levels of it are known to decrease in winter when there is less natural exposure to sunlight. Although vitamin D is found in oily fish and eggs, it can be difficult to obtain the sufficient amount, so taking a supplement will help to increase your levels.

Warning

According to the Food Standards Agency, women who are planning a pregnancy should not eat more than two servings of tinned tuna a week, because of the risk of mercury contamination.

18. Try natural sperm boosters

Making some simple dietary changes to improve your partner's sperm before you try to conceive is worthwhile, as it will benefit his overall health. Remember, sperm takes 100 days to develop, 74 days to form and 20–30 days to mature, so try and include the following foods three months before trying for a baby.

Essential fatty acids

EFAs act as hormone regulators; men who are deficient in EFAs will have poor-quality sperm with a low count and may even have abnormal sperm. You can get EFAs from linseeds, oily fish, such as salmon, herrings, mackerel, trout and sardines, green leafy vegetables and walnuts. EFA supplements are screened for toxins and purified.

Protein

Protein contains the amino acids, especially L-arginine, L-carnitine and taurine, required to make healthy sperm. Research has shown that sperm counts doubled after protein supplements were taken. Arginine supplements should not be taken by men who suffer from the herpes virus, as it can stimulate an attack.

Vitamin A

This vitamin is essential for the male reproductive system and production of male sex hormones. The recommended amount for men is 700 micrograms (mcg) per day.

Folic acid

Folate (folic acid) improves sperm motility and sperm count and research has shown it is just as important for men as for women.

Warning

Liver is rich in folic acid, but women planning to become pregnant or who are pregnant should not eat it as it is high in vitamin A. High levels of vitamin A may harm your unborn baby.

Vitamin B6

Essential for the production of male sex hormones, studies have shown that a vitamin B6 deficiency in animals causes infertility.

Vitamin B12

Low levels of B12 are linked to reduced sperm count, abnormal sperm and reduced sperm motility.

Vitamin C

Vitamin C improves motility and sperm count and prevents the clumping together of the sperm. Research has shown that men with low vitamin C levels were more likely to have genetically damaged sperm.

Vitamin E

Vitamin E is needed for healthy sperm and is thought to improve a sperm's ability to penetrate an egg.

Selenium

Selenium is necessary for the formation of sperm and for a good sperm count. Low levels of selenium are linked to infertility in men.

Zinc

Zinc is vital for the production of healthy sperm but is often missing from modern diets. Research shows that supplementing zinc improves fertility.

19. Consult a nutritionist

Nutrition consultant and author Ian Marber, known as the 'Food Doctor', believes fertility problems have increased dramatically over the last 20 years for both men and women. He recommends that couples should eat a healthy balanced diet of organic fruit, vegetables and meat and that men should increase their intake of food rich in zinc, such as shellfish, nuts and seeds, in particular pumpkin seeds. He also recommends that, to improve their fertility, women should eat foods high in vitamin B6, like watercress, peppers, asparagus, chicken, eggs, lentils and brown rice. Marber emphasises the importance of steering clear of convenience foods and foods high in sugar, replacing sugary snacks with fresh fruit and avoiding caffeine. He also advocates drinking at least one litre of water a day. Nutritional therapist Dr Marilyn Glenville also emphasises the importance of a healthy diet for a successful pregnancy and to help with hormonal imbalances that may affect fertility.

The fertility diet in a nutshell

A balanced diet containing whole grains, oats, pulses, linseed oil, fresh fruit, vegetables, oily fish, shellfish, nuts and seeds, eggs, chicken, olive oil and plenty of water will help to supply the nutrients required for fertility.

Chapter 3

Natural Ways to Improve Your Fertility

We've already looked at the importance of a healthy diet and how an unbalanced diet can affect fertility in both men and women. This chapter discusses natural ways to give your fertility a boost, including taking herbal, vitamin and mineral supplements.

20. Take supplements

According to research, supplements are growing in popularity and studies have shown that couples who take supplements over a 14-month period conceive earlier than those not taking them. While supplements are often controversial, as some experts believe that a healthy diet should provide all the nutrients you require for a healthy body, many of us recognise that supplements offer a convenient way of ensuring we receive the required amount of vitamins and minerals. Midwives, health visitors and other health experts may recommend some of the supplements especially produced for preconception healthcare. In April 2010, the *British Journal of Nutrition* published a randomised, double-blind, placebo-controlled trial of a multiple micronutrient supplement that may improve the health of pregnant women and their babies. Their findings showed that significant levels of mineral and vitamin deficiency amongst mothers during early pregnancy were significantly improved in the third trimester (weeks 29–40) after supplementation. It doesn't mean that all supplements are as effective: sometimes the research gives results that are deemed inconclusive, especially if the study is not carried out scientifically. Also, some herbal remedies have several active ingredients and this can make it difficult to pinpoint the ones that are beneficial. The quality of herbal remedies can also differ according to the type of soil they are grown in and the methods of extraction, storage, production etc., making firm conclusions regarding particular herbs difficult.

Safe supplements

There is a Traditional Herbal Medicines Registration Scheme under which herbal products in the UK are now registered, but some still remain unregistered. From April 2011, all herbal medicines are required to have either a traditional herbal medicine registration or a product licence.

It is worth remembering that it can be counterproductive to take too much of a mineral or vitamin: high doses of one can affect the levels of another. It is best to consult a nutritionist and, if you do take supplements, ensure you stick to the recommended dosages.

Listed below are a range of commercial formulations currently available from chemists, supermarkets and health food shops and online.

Conception and Wellman Conception are a range of fertility and conception supplements that provide nutritional support when planning a baby and after you've conceived. They include a his and her conception dual pack, with vitamin B12, L-arginine and folic acid for women, and folic acid, coenzyme Q10 and lycopene for men.

Mumomega is a supplement containing omega-3 fatty acids, including DHA-rich marine fish oil, omega-6 and vitamin E that can be taken before, during and after pregnancy. It also contains virgin evening primrose oil.

Folic acid tablets are available from many chemists and supermarkets. Look for formulas that supply the recommended daily amount (400 mcg). These tablets should be taken before pregnancy and for the first 12 weeks after conception.

Vitabiotics Pregnacare Plus with omega-3 contains 17 nutrients, including B12 and folic acid at the recommended daily dosage along with omega-3 fatty acids, DHA and EPA and can be taken before, during and after pregnancy.

Sanatogen mother to be and Sanatogen father to be are two different multivitamin and multi-mineral supplements, with zinc for men and folic acid for women, and are suitable for couples trying for a baby.

Prebio 7 is a probiotic supplement containing two types of fibre and seven types of friendly bacteria thought to optimise the levels of intestinal flora essential for good health and vitality. It can be taken by both men and women before pregnancy.

Babystart has a range of supplements to assist conception for women and men. All their products are environmentally friendly.

Zita West has a range of fertility supplements available from her clinic or online, for men and women, which can be taken before, during and after pregnancy. Her details can be found in the Directory at the back of the book.

Dr Marilyn Glenville has developed Fertility Plus for Women and Fertility Plus for Men, which include the amino acids L-arginine, L-carnitine and L-taurine. Her details are in the Directory. These supplements can be taken to increase the chances of conception either naturally or by IVF treatment.

21. Benefit from herbs

Various herbs have been used throughout the centuries to help fertility and conception. Because they are totally natural, they are becoming popular fertility options. Of course, it is best to seek help from a qualified practitioner rather than self-treat or self-diagnose; just because herbs may be natural doesn't mean they are safe. The National Institute of Medical Herbalists, listed in the Directory at the back of the book, will help you find a qualified practitioner in your area who will prescribe herbs to work in cooperation with your body.

Word of warning

Do not take any herbs if you are taking the contraceptive pill, fertility drugs such as clomid, or having assisted conception treatment such as IVF, unless prescribed by a qualified practitioner.

Safety first

Always buy your herbs from a reputable company. The government's Medicines and Healthcare Products Regulatory Agency offers further advice about using herbal medicines safely. The contact details are in the Directory.

Agnus castus

Also known as chaste tree berry or vitex, this is a shrub native to West Asia and south-western Europe and was introduced to England in the sixteenth century. It is the first-choice herb for increasing fertility, balancing hormones and encouraging ovulation. In one study, 48 women diagnosed with infertility took Agnus castus daily for three months, seven of them became pregnant within that time and 25 of them regained normal progesterone levels. This herb is thought to be very beneficial for women with a short second luteal phase of their monthly cycle and it also helps to lower high prolactin levels, which are known to cause infertility. It is known to act directly on the pituitary gland, which, amongst other things, is responsible for the FSH and LH. It can be taken in pill or tincture form.

Black cohosh

Black cohosh is a member of the buttercup family and is found in North America, where it is widely used by native Americans to treat gynaecological problems. It stimulates the release of LH, and contains isoflavone constituents that have oestrogen-like properties. It is safest when taken in a herbal formula prescribed by a qualified herbalist and should not be taken during pregnancy.

Dong quai

This herb is native to China and is used to strengthen a weak uterus and regulate hormones and the menstrual cycle. However, it must be taken under supervision as it contains micronutrients known for their blood-building properties. It is also a blood-thinner and can cause heavy bleeding during periods. It should not be taken with anti-coagulant drugs.

Evening primrose oil

Evening primrose oil is in omega-3 and is often found in commercial supplement formulations. It is thought to help increase fertile cervical fluid and can be taken in herbal form from menstruation to ovulation. After ovulation, herbalists suggest switching to flaxseed oil as it may cause uterine contractions. It can be taken in liquid or capsule form.

False unicorn root

False unicorn root is used for amenorrhoea (reduced or non-existent periods), hormonal balance and infertility. It is a tonic for the female reproductive organs and is thought to support the normal functioning of the ovaries. It is also said to be helpful to men with a low sperm count and motility. It can be taken in tincture, tea or tablet form.

Liquorice

Liquorice can help women who have irregular periods and those with low levels of oestrogen and high levels of testosterone. It is another herb that should be taken under supervision as it has a high sodium content and may not be suitable for those with high blood pressure or kidney problems. It can be taken as a tincture, or in tea or pill form, or by chewing the root.

Motherwort

Motherwort is a member of the mint family. Originally from Central Asia, it is now used worldwide as a uterine tonic, a type of herbal remedy that is known to strengthen the female reproductive system. It can be taken in tincture or tablet form.

Pycnogenol

This natural plant extract, originating from the bark of the maritime pine that grows along the coast of south-west France, acts as an antioxidant and is considered to help increase normal-functioning sperm. According to a study published in the October 2002 issue of the *Journal of Reproductive Medicine*, the quality and function of sperm of men with fertility problems who used this plant extract for 90 days improved by 38 per cent and 19 per cent respectively. It can be taken in tablet or tincture form, and is suitable for both men and women.

Red clover

Red clover is known to have oestrogen-like compounds and is thought to aid the uterus. It can be taken in tincture, tea or tablet form, and is suitable for both men and women.

Saw Palmetto

Saw Palmetto is a natural steroid-source herb with tissue-building and gland-stimulating properties to strengthen and tone the male reproductive system. It is thought to help men with low libido and promote prostate health. It can be taken in tincture, tea or tablet form, and is suitable for both men and women.

Siberian ginseng

This herb is thought to help the body cope better with stress and support the adrenal glands. It is available as a tea, as well as in tincture and pill form.

Wild yam

Wild yam is thought to increase progesterone production and can be used by those with short luteal phases, but it should only be taken after ovulation because, if it is taken before, it can actually prevent ovulation. It can be taken in tincture or pill form.

Herbs to avoid

The following herbs are thought to have a negative effect on fertility: burdock, catnip, celery seed, camomile, cohosh, fennel, juniper, pennyroyal and sage. According to a recent study, St John's wort, gingko biloba and Echinacea reduce sperm quality and the ability to penetrate an egg.

Chapter 4

Preparing for Conception

All fertility experts agree that preparing both you and your partner for conception and pregnancy at least three months before you plan to start a family is beneficial. This way you can both ensure you are in the best possible health, mentally and physically.

We have already seen how diet and nutrients affect conception and regulate the sex hormones, ovulation, regular monthly cycles and sperm production. This chapter looks at evaluating your fertility before you begin to try to conceive and the importance of planning ahead for a baby, such as stopping smoking and watching your weight. It also stresses the importance of regular exercise and getting enough sleep.

The effects of stress are examined and details are given on the techniques and methods you can use to help you deal with it more effectively. It also provides information on limiting your daily exposure to environmental toxins.

Where do you stand?
There are so many factors that affect fertility that taking stock of where you stand at the moment, how your health is, whether your diet is healthy and whether you need to make any lifestyle changes before embarking on trying for a baby, will be worthwhile in the long run. Many fertility specialists will consider a list of points before

trying to help you diagnose any fertility issues or potential fertility problems. However, should you feel you already have a fertility problem consult your doctor immediately so that he or she can help and can begin the testing process.

Fertility checklist

The list below will help you to identify your next move or any changes you might need to make in order to give you the best possible chance to get pregnant.

◯ Age: the older you are, the less fertile you are. If you are 35 or over, consider seeking professional advice if you have not conceived after having regular unprotected sex for six months.

◯ Your contraceptive history: contraceptive methods used in the past may have affected your fertility. Women who have used the contraceptive pill may not understand their monthly cycle or the best time to conceive. Ask your doctor for help should this be the case or if you suspect any damage from previous contraception, such an infection from an intra-uterine device.

◯ Weight: your weight needs to be within the recommended BMI. See further on in this chapter for more information.

◯ Your menstrual cycle: is your menstrual cycle regular and do you understand when ovulation should occur? If you are unsure, consider seeking fertility advice from a fertility counsellor.

◯ Family history: are there any genetic problems you may have inherited? Check with your family and your partner's family to see if there might be anything that could affect your fertility.

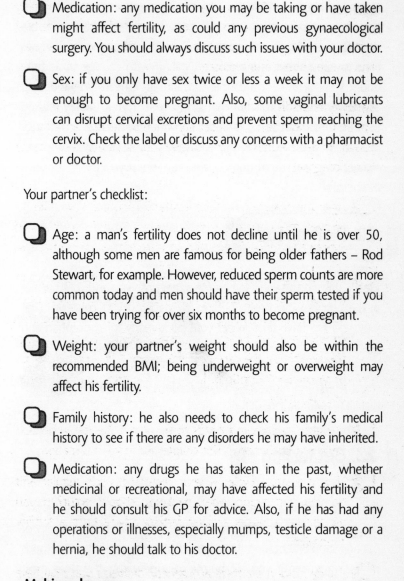

Medication: any medication you may be taking or have taken might affect fertility, as could any previous gynaecological surgery. You should always discuss such issues with your doctor.

Sex: if you only have sex twice or less a week it may not be enough to become pregnant. Also, some vaginal lubricants can disrupt cervical excretions and prevent sperm reaching the cervix. Check the label or discuss any concerns with a pharmacist or doctor.

Your partner's checklist:

Age: a man's fertility does not decline until he is over 50, although some men are famous for being older fathers – Rod Stewart, for example. However, reduced sperm counts are more common today and men should have their sperm tested if you have been trying for over six months to become pregnant.

Weight: your partner's weight should also be within the recommended BMI; being underweight or overweight may affect his fertility.

Family history: he also needs to check his family's medical history to see if there are any disorders he may have inherited.

Medication: any drugs he has taken in the past, whether medicinal or recreational, may have affected his fertility and he should consult his GP for advice. Also, if he has had any operations or illnesses, especially mumps, testicle damage or a hernia, he should talk to his doctor.

Making changes
Very often couples can be worried about others and what they think as they make the necessary changes to their lifestyles and diet

to aid fertility. Some may be wary of comments from friends when they give up smoking or alcohol, others may feel that people are waiting for them to announce news of their pregnancy, which can lead to extra stress and tension. Dealing with change takes time and it's important for a couple to maintain a healthy relationship as they embark on this life-changing event. Trying to stay relaxed may be difficult at times, and sex can often be seen as a necessity instead of a pleasurable and fun occasion. Communicating and maintaining a sense of humour and fun whilst you try to conceive are helpful.

22. Plan ahead

Ideally, it is worth taking some time to get both you and your partner in the best possible health before you start to try to conceive. That way, you will have time to get your body ready for conception and give yourself the best possible chance. Checking your diet for any nutritional deficiencies, losing weight if necessary, reducing your stress levels and reducing your exposure to environmental hazards will all benefit your fertility.

23. Get testing

Seeing a nutritional therapist is a way of ensuring you are getting the most from your diet and whether you may need vitamin or mineral supplementation. However, there are several other methods of testing to see if you are nutritionally deficient; the three most common tests are listed below. Very often, a nutritionist will suggest using them as part of his or her screening process.

Hair analysis

Whilst there is a lot of debate among health professionals about the usefulness of hair analysis, Foresight has been using it for over 30 years to determine mineral and heavy metal toxicity status. Hair cells are the fastest-growing cells in the body; as they grow, they lock in the nutrients and toxins you have been exposed to. Levels of essential nutrients, such as magnesium, calcium, zinc, selenium, copper, manganese and chromium can be assessed, as well as harmful toxins including lead, aluminium, cadmium and mercury. A qualified practitioner can then decide the levels of vitamins and minerals you need to correct any deficiencies and cleanse any toxins from your body.

Saliva test

A saliva test can determine your levels of oestrogen and progesterone. There are several types of saliva tests available at chemists and online that you can use at home.

Iridology

Iridology is an alternative medicine technique whose followers believe that the patterns, colours, lines and markings of the iris can be examined to determine a patient's systemic health. Practitioners match their observations to iris charts, which divide the iris into zones that correspond to specific parts of the body. It is a non-invasive test that is thought to reveal vitamin and mineral deficiencies as well as allergies and hormonal imbalance.

24. Stop smoking

The health hazards of smoking, such as lung cancer and emphysema, are well documented, but it's not often that couples realise just what an effect smoking has on their fertility. Smoking damages the ovaries, increases the risk of cervical cancer, causes hormonal changes and, in some cases, can bring on early menopause, which can be devastating if you are considering conceiving at a later stage in life. According to the *British Medical Journal*, women who smoke reduce their probability of conceiving naturally, and increase the risk of IVF failure, while approximately 120,000 men aged between 30 and 50 are impotent as a result of smoking.

Smoking damages a man's sperm, lowers sperm count and can lead to impotence by damaging the blood vessels and reducing blood flow to the testicles. Studies suggest male smokers are at least 50 per cent more likely to suffer from erectile dysfunction.

It may be difficult to quit, but there is plenty of help and support available – see your GP for details of your nearest smoking cessation clinic. Alternatively, visit www.smokefree.nhs.uk or call the free NHS Smoking Helpline on 0800 022 4332 for information about the free NHS services available to help you stop smoking. Giving up before you conceive will also benefit your unborn baby.

25. Cut the caffeine

Caffeine robs the body of important vitamins and minerals and increases the stress hormone cortisol, which depletes the adrenal glands. This competes with progesterone and can lead to oestrogen dominance and a hormonal imbalance, and is known to reduce both men's and women's fertility and ability to conceive. If your partner is suffering with sperm problems, such as a low sperm count, caffeine can exacerbate the problem; it is thought to negate vital nutrients, like zinc, that are important for fertility.

According to one study, drinking or eating moderate amounts of caffeine is thought to lower your fertility by as much as 27 per cent (moderate amounts of caffeine in this study were two cups of coffee, four cups of tea or five cans of cola per day, or approximately 200 mg). It is thought that caffeine reduces your chance of conceiving if you are having IVF treatment and it's worth remembering that caffeine is not just found in coffee, tea and cola: it is also an ingredient in other soft drinks, chocolate and even some prescribed medication. Try replacing caffeine with herbal teas, redbush tea and water. Many fertility experts advise you not to drink decaffeinated drinks, as they may contain other harmful ingredients.

Caffeine content of drinks/foods

Food/drink	Approximate caffeine content (mg)
Ground coffee (cup)	110
Instant coffee (cup)	60
Painkillers (two tablets)	60
Tea (cup)	50
Cola (one can)	40
Milk chocolate (125 g/4 oz bar)	20
Cocoa (cup)	5

26. Replace bad fats

Saturated fat is solid at room temperature and is found in animal products, such as red meat (it is the white skin you see on red meat) and full-fat dairy products (butter, cheese and whole milk), as well as biscuits, cakes and sweets. All of these products are known to stimulate oestrogen production and can compromise your fertility.

Eating too much saturated fat is known to increase cholesterol levels and the risk of heart disease, obesity and certain types of cancer, so it really is worthwhile to limit your intake. See Chapter 2 for information on good fats.

27. Detox your body

The liver is the detoxifying organ of the body, ridding it of caffeine, alcohol, drugs, pesticides, food additives and preservatives and environmental toxins like petrol fumes and tobacco smoke. It also produces substances to break down fats and chemically alters hormones so they can either be re-circulated or excreted. The hormonal balance required for fertility relies on good liver function. Some fertility experts believe the liver should be given periods of detoxification by eating only foods that it does not have to work too hard to break down. The length of detoxification varies: Zita West suggests a liver detox of seven to ten days. However, if you are on medication, consult your doctor beforehand and also stop the programme if you experience any pain or discomfort.

Foods to limit
By reducing your intake of certain foods in the first few days, you may find you experience a few withdrawal headaches, but these should soon pass. The foods to restrict include alcohol, red meat, caffeine, wheat and dairy products.

Foods to aid liver function

Fruit and vegetables aid the liver; increasing your intake of these foods will increase your natural fibre content.

- Apples contain pectin, which is thought to bind and excrete heavy metals, reducing the filtration the liver carries out.

- Garlic contains allicin, an antioxidant, and selenium. It also assists the removal of heavy metals from the liver.

- Carrots, red onions, beetroot and aubergine contain the antioxidants flavonoids and beta-carotene.

- Cruciferous vegetables such as cauliflower, broccoli, cabbage and lettuce contain glucosinolates, which help the liver produce enzymes for detoxification.

- Eggs, brown rice, whole grains, spinach and broccoli all contain B vitamins, which improve liver function and promote liver decongestion. Vitamin B12 helps improve liver health.

Supplements to support your liver

You can take a herbal supplement to support your liver during the detoxification process. Expert advice is divided over whether or not nutritional supplements are a necessary addition to a detox diet. Many detox nutritional supplements contain a range of natural ingredients, including prebiotics and milk thistle. Silymarin is a milk thistle extract and clinical trials have proved the efficiency of this herb for liver disorders.

Listed below is a range of commercial formulations currently available from chemists, supermarkets, health food shops and online.

Wellwoman Inner Cleanse – This food supplement provides dietary support while detoxing. It provides 26 vitamins, minerals and other nutrients, including amino acids, vitamin E, dandelion root, grapefruit extract and artichoke, to help maintain a strong immune system and eliminate impurities.

Boots Milk Thistle Tincture – Boots Milk Thistle Tincture contains seeds of the plant Silybum marianum. It is taken in water or with juice three times a day.

Duchy Herbals Detox Tincture – This food supplement is made from extracts of artichoke and dandelion, which are cleansing and purifying herbs that help support the body's natural elimination and detoxification processes and aid digestion.

Detox precautions

1. If you are taking any form of medication, check with your doctor before embarking on a detox programme.
2. It is best to seek advice from a qualified nutritionist about a detox programme.
3. Do not attempt exercise whilst on a detox programme.
4. Ensure you get plenty of rest whilst detoxing.
5. Do not start a detox if you are already under a lot of stress.
6. If you feel very ill or experience pain, stop the detox.
7. During the early stages of a detox you may experience headaches.

28. Moderate your alcohol intake

There is evidence to support the belief that alcohol directly affects the fertility of both men and women. In males, it decreases sperm count, increases abnormal sperm and affects hormone levels, which suppresses production of testosterone, decreases libido and can cause impotence. Alcohol also affects the absorption of zinc, which is vital for male fertility: it not only makes the tail and outer layer of the sperm, but low levels of zinc reduce sperm count.

Alcohol has a more systemic response on females, affecting the reproductive hormones and leading to abnormalities in the menstrual cycle. The *British Medical Journal* published research data suggesting that women who drank socially, i.e. one to five units per week, were at a greater risk of being unable to conceive compared to women who did not drink. Another study showed that women who drank less than five units a week (equivalent to five standard pub measures: 50 ml of wine or 25 ml of spirits), were twice as likely to conceive within six months compared to those who drank more. Experts suggest cutting back or giving up alcohol completely for three months before trying to conceive.

29. Watch your weight

There is evidence to show that being underweight or overweight will affect your fertility, as both disrupt your hormonal balance. Body mass index (BMI) is the standard measure to assess whether you are under or over your ideal weight. There is a strong link between having a high BMI and PCOS, menstrual irregularities and ovulation infrequency. Women with a high BMI may have a significantly lower chance of success with IVF or intra-uterine insemination treatment. Being underweight makes conception difficult as well, as this may disrupt hormones and lead to infrequent or suppressed ovulation.

Calculate your BMI

Calculating your BMI will determine if you are a healthy weight.

1. Work out your height in metres and multiply the figure by itself. This is your height squared.

2. Measure your weight in kilograms.

3. Divide your weight by your height squared.

For example, here is the calculation for a person who is 1.6 m tall and weighs 65 kg :
1.6 x 1.6 = 2.56
65 divided by 2.56 = 25.39

A BMI of between 18.5 and 24.9 indicates a healthy weight. Below 18.5 is classed as underweight, while anything above 24.9 is deemed overweight. A BMI of 30 or more is considered obese. Bear in mind that body frames vary and it's more accurate to recommend a weight range rather than a specific weight for a given height.

Obesity and fertility

The British Fertility Society advises obese women to start weight loss programmes before treating them, to improve their chances of getting pregnant. Researchers also discovered that obese men produce 60 per cent less seminal fluid than men with a healthy BMI, and had 40 per cent higher levels of abnormal sperm. And in another study, researchers found that diabetes, which is closely linked to obesity, also damages fertility.

30. Take a little exercise every day

Exercise is essential as part of a healthy lifestyle and, when pursued in moderation, can actually help to increase your fertility. In the UK, most people's lifestyles are increasingly sedentary, fewer people walk or cycle on a daily basis and modern living and desk-bound jobs have us all sitting for longer periods of the day and evening than ever before. Yet research shows that, along with a healthy diet, exercise can stimulate fertility and may help you to conceive.

Regular exercise can lead to a healthier body, reduce stress, help you lose weight and boost your self-esteem, while endorphins released during exercise produce the hormone serotonin, making you feel happier.

Being active is not all about going to the gym or running outside in the freezing cold in shorts: it's much simpler and easier than that. Generally, physical activity is any exercise that raises your heart rate and any moderate activity that you enjoy and fits into your lifestyle will improve your well-being.

There are plenty of simple ways to become more active on a daily basis: using the stairs instead of the lift, swimming, cycling or brisk walking are all ideal.

The benefits of regular exercise

Regular exercise has a wide range of benefits, including:

- Making you physically fitter
- Improving your mental health
- Improving your immune system
- Improving your sense of well-being and making you feel happier
- Reducing your stress levels
- Aiding sleep

Reducing the risk of heart disease, stroke, diabetes and obesity

Reducing the risk of some types of cancer

Helping to reduce blood pressure

Releasing endorphins

How much?

According to the Department of Health, the current recommendations for the general health of adults is a minimum of 30 minutes of moderate physical activity on at least five days of the week. This can be achieved in bouts of 10 minutes or more over the course of the day. This can include walking or cycling for all or part of your journey to work; doing manual tasks or using the stairs.

However, your routine could include two to three more intense sessions, which you could consider doing at the weekend such as running, cycling, swimming, tennis, squash or badminton, or something simple like taking a long walk, gardening or a session at the gym.

If you are overweight, the Department of Health recommends 45–60 minutes of exercise a day with a change to your diet. Even brisk walking for this length of time with a controlled diet will ensure weight loss. See NHS Inform (www.nhsinform.co.uk) for further information.

What works?

All exercise is good for you, and the best forms of exercise are those that you enjoy doing and those that fit easily into your daily routine. It is much more beneficial to make sure you have some form of exercise every day than it is to overexert yourself for longer periods twice a week. The Change4Life website (www.nhs.uk/change4life) has some interesting ideas and suggestions for helping you to get active.

Types of exercise

Aerobic exercise, such as an instructor-led aerobics class, jogging or swimming, will raise your heart rate and improve your strength and stamina. They are good for your heart, general health and your circulation (your reproductive organs require a healthy blood flow) and will help you to burn fat and lose weight if combined with a sensible healthy eating plan.

Strength training requires short bursts of activity and energy and will burn calories, improve posture, balance and stability, and strengthen your bones. Pilates and yoga are good examples of strength training. Stretching or flexibility exercises help to reduce muscle tension and improve flexibility and posture. They are all useful for preparing the body for pregnancy.

Too much exercise

Studies have shown that excessive aerobic exercise can have adverse effects on fertility. Excessive exercise for men may reduce sperm count, as it can lead to the testicles overheating, while women's fertility may be compromised if they lose too much body fat, as this reduces oestrogen and increases the risk of irregular ovulation.

Exercise safely

If you have any health concerns, see your GP before embarking on a fitness regime.

---

31. Get outside

Being outside in natural sunlight is thought to benefit ovulation and the reproductive hormones in both men and women, aiding the production of testosterone in males and directly affecting ovulation and reproductive hormones.

Some fertility experts believe that depression caused by a lack of natural sunlight, better known as Seasonal Affective Disorder (SAD), can suppress fertility as it affects both sleep and mood. Bright light is also thought to help fertility by correcting menstrual irregularities, and the therapeutic use of bright light to restore fertility is under investigation.

Researchers have discovered that pregnancy from IVF is more likely between May and September: fewer drugs are required to stimulate ovulation in women during the months with the most sunlight and success rates increase in the lighter months.

Researchers also found that decreased levels of vitamin D, which are a problem for many people during the winter months when there is less exposure to natural sunlight, produced problems with ovulation.

According to the British Association of Dermatologists, the amount of time you need to spend in the sun to make enough vitamin D varies from person to person, and depends on other factors such as your skin type, your geographical location, the time of day and even the time of year, so there is some confusion over exposing your skin safely without getting burnt. It is thought that spending ten minutes a day in natural sunlight will help to boost your vitamin D levels. Simply going for a quick stroll around your garden or down to the shops can be beneficial.

Stay safe in the sun

The current advice from Cancer Research UK advises the following for adults:

- Seek out shade between 11 a.m. and 3 p.m.
- Cover up with clothing, a hat and sunglasses.
- Use factor 15 sunscreen or higher.

32. Ditch the drugs

Even the occasional recreational drug can play havoc with fertility, affecting your hormone production, cervical mucus and ovulation. Cannabis, for example, will affect a man's sperm production and lower his libido. However, certain over-the-counter drugs and prescription drugs such as antibiotics can also affect your fertility, so make sure you tell your doctor if you are taking prescription drugs and are trying to conceive.

33. Keep him cool

The male reproductive organs are on the outside of the body and need to be kept several degrees cooler than normal body temperature, as sperm production can only take place at 32°C (89°F) – normal body temperature is 37°C (98.4°F). If the testes are heated up, the sperm count can be decreased. Research has shown that an increase of even 1°C in testicular or scrotal temperature can decrease the production of healthy sperm by as much as 40 per cent. Men should avoid wearing tight underpants or trousers, should take showers instead of hot baths, avoid crossing their legs and make sure they get up frequently and move around, especially if their job involves sitting down for long periods.

It's also a good idea not to use an electric blanket in bed: not only will it provide too much heat to a man's testicles, but it also emits electromagnetic radiation, another potential fertility hazard.

> ### Laptops on laps
>
> A recent study from researchers at the State University of New York found that men who regularly balance their laptops on their laps when working may be jeopardising their ability to have children. The risk comes from the heat generated from the laptop computer to the scrotum, heating the testicles and causing testicular dysfunction.

34. Sleep soundly

The quantity and quality of your sleep is thought to affect your fertility, health, hormones and mood. Sleep helps to restore the body and insufficient sleep can disrupt oestrogen, progesterone, lutenising hormone, follicle-stimulating hormone and leptin, which affects ovulation. Lack of sleep may also lead to fertility-disrupting lifestyle factors like caffeine overuse and weight gain and menstrual and ovulation irregularities. Studies have shown that women whose work involves shift patterns or deprived sleep situations, such as flight stewardesses, are more than likely to have an irregular menstrual cycle.

Stress can also affect fertility, and people who suffer from chronic stress often find their sleeping habits affected. Feelings of anxiety and depression can arise and studies have shown that fertility patients have lower IVF success rates if they are suffering from anxiety and depression. The levels of the stress hormone cortisol rise as stress increases, affecting progesterone levels, which in turn affect fertility. Exposure to artificial light from computers, light bulbs, television and electronic games can also inhibit sleep.

To sleep more soundly, try the following:

1. Be consistent in your bedtime routine. Go to bed at the same time each night and get up at the same time, even at weekends and during holidays.

2. Avoid coffee, cigarettes and alcohol, all of which are negative influences on your fertility anyway.

3. Exercise daily, but not too close to bedtime.

4. Try to get outside every day.

5. See your doctor if your sleep pattern is badly affected.

If you are having trouble sleeping, try the Sleep Council (www.sleepcouncil.com) for support and advice. The Royal College of Psychiatrists has an excellent leaflet on sleeping well that contains tips and ideas on getting a good night's sleep (www.rcpsych.ac.uk).

35. Have happy sex

Research has shown that women who have happy and enjoyable sex and have orgasms retain more sperm than those who don't, as muscular contractions during orgasm help to propel the sperm towards the uterus.

Any which way
According to Professor Ledger, Professor of Obstetrics and Gynaecology at the University of Sheffield, there are no particular positions that guarantee conception. However, other fertility experts disagree and believe the missionary position, where the man is on top, is one of the best ways to help conception, as it

allows the deepest penetration, with the sperm being deposited next to the cervix. The man penetrating the women from behind is another position that may also aid conception as it also allows the sperm to be deposited right next to the opening of the womb. The old wives' tale of raising your legs above your hips or up against the wall is also thought to encourage the sperm to swim the right way up the Fallopian tubes.

Stay in bed
Don't leap out of bed straight after sex. Instead, lie on your side and place a pillow under your hips and relax for a while.

A touch of romance

Book a weekend break or a romantic dinner for two to ensure the romance in your life continues. This can be particularly important if you have been trying for a baby for some time and sex has become a scheduled, planned 'must-do-it-now' activity. Taking time out for just the two of you will help you both relax and may even boost libido.

36. Seek help

Sometimes, no matter how much you try, getting pregnant just does not happen. If you and your partner have been having unprotected sex for a year or over and are under 30 years of age, seek advice from your doctor, who will offer you fertility testing. If you are over 35, fertility experts agree that if you have not fallen pregnant after six months of unprotected intercourse, you should see your doctor and ask for fertility tests.

Should you embark on fertility testing, it is worth discussing your course of action with your partner so that you can support each other during the testing time. Each test will determine the next course of action, so try not to have fixed ideas about what is going to happen.

It is worthwhile getting your partner to have his sperm tested at the same time as you start your fertility tests as a man's fertility can be the obstacle preventing conception in 20 per cent of cases. It is a non-invasive and relatively simple test that can often lead to identifying the problem that, with treatment, can very often result in a successful pregnancy.

37. Test for STIs

Sexually transmitted infections (STIs) can seriously damage your fertility. STIs are passed on through intimate sexual contact and common ones include chlamydia and gonorrhoea. According to the Health Protection Agency, STIs are on the increase in the UK, so if you or your partner has had unprotected sex in the past it is worthwhile getting yourselves tested at your local family planning clinic. See Chapter 5 for more information on STIs.

38. Understand and manage stress

Stress is the body's way of responding to any kind of demand, either emotional or physical, that leaves us feeling unable to cope or inadequate. It can vary from person to person; one person may cope well in a particular situation while another finds the same situation stressful – it all comes down to the individual's perception and ability to deal with it.

How stress affects the body

Whenever the body reacts to a situation, it releases the hormones cortisol, adrenaline and noradrenaline into the bloodstream. The brain reacts by preparing the body to either stay and face the perceived threat or to take flight and escape from it. This 'fight or flight' response is known as survival stress and is a common response in all people. Today, most stressful situations are considered to be internal, and those that continue for a long time with no end in sight, such as divorce, illness, money worries or long-term unemployment, mean that stress levels remain high, increasing blood pressure and the risk of major health conditions like heart attacks. It also has a direct effect on fertility by affecting the hormones that govern the production of eggs and testosterone.

Stress and your fertility

According to research, psychological treatment to relieve stress can achieve excellent results, restoring fertility to women who do not ovulate or menstruate. The findings suggest that using stress-reducing techniques can be the most effective way of treating amenorrhoea (lack of periods), which affects up to one in ten women of reproductive age.

Other research has found that reducing stress during IVF treatment can dramatically improve the chances of success.

How to recognise stress

If you are under stress, changes in your cervical mucus may indicate something is wrong. As you approach ovulation, increased cervical wetness may be interspersed with dry days and, unless you are using a method of ovulation detection such as plotting your temperature or using an ovulation predictor test, you may not notice you have ovulated. Although stress-induced delays to ovulation should not stop you getting pregnant if you are having sex every two to three days throughout your cycle, your stress and anxiety may mean you are having less sex than this and you miss the opportunity to conceive. If you have stopped ovulating because of stress, you may need hormone therapy or cognitive behaviour therapy (changing the way you think and the way you deal with stress).

Simple self-help stress techniques

There are a number of ways to help you deal with everyday stress. The list below offers some simple ideas:

- Exercise regularly to release endorphins to improve your general health and sense of well-being.

- Make time to meditate – a simple meditation can help you overcome stress. Learn to transform negative thoughts to positive ones, which will leave you feeling calmer and more focused. The effects of meditation are more noticeable when it is done consistently and regularly. You can learn meditation techniques by using CDs or DVDs or by going to a meditation class.

- Deep breathing techniques are known to help you relax. When you breathe deeply, your lungs fill with more oxygen, which helps to reduce tension and anxiety. Here is a simple breathing exercise: sit comfortably, with your back straight, or lie on the floor on your back. Place your hands on your stomach and breathe in through your nose for a count of eight. Feel your hands rise on your stomach. Breathe out gently through your mouth for a count of eight. Practise breathing like this every day for ten minutes or so.

Try yoga – one of the most ancient forms of exercise and relaxation – to improve muscle tone and strength through different postures and breathing. See Chapter 7 for the suggested yoga poses you can try for boosting fertility. The best way to enjoy and learn yoga is to attend a class run by a qualified practitioner. The British Wheel of Yoga (www.bwy.org.uk) will help you find a class in your area. If you wish to practise it at home, there are plenty of yoga DVDs to rent or buy. You can always try YouTube (www.youtube.com) for some yoga postures, but do take care when trying postures you are not familiar with.

39. Limit your exposure to environmental toxins

There is now a substantial amount of research to indicate that certain heavy metals circulating in the body can interfere with fertility. Toxins are everywhere: in the air, the water, food, homes and toiletries. Many of these toxins not only adversely affect our general health but they can also impair fertility. Daily contact with chemicals from household cleaners, aerosols, deodorants, hairspray, perfume and even shower gels accumulate in the cells of our bodies over time, while exposure to heavy metals, including lead from petrol fumes, mercury from dental fillings and oily fish, aluminium in foil, cookware, canned drinks and deodorants, and cadmium in cigarette smoke, all have a negative effect on egg and sperm production and sperm quality. Heavy metal toxicity may result in fatigue, damaged or reduced central nervous function and damage to organs. They may also cause allergies.

Xenoestrogens, oestrogen-like chemicals in the environment resulting from pollution from the manufacture of plastics and pesticides, are known to affect the reproductive hormones, whilst dioxins and polychlorinated biphenyls found in soil and the water are passed into milk, meat, eggs and fish. Lord Professor Robert Winston, a leading UK fertility expert, advised against wearing perfume or aftershave in order to avoid chemicals when trying to maximise fertility.

Recent surveys have shown that some fish contain dioxins and polychlorinated biphenyls. They include brown crabmeat, sea bream, sea bass, turbot, halibut and rock salmon.

The Food Standards Agency advises the following when choosing seafood:

◖ Select fish and shellfish from responsibly managed sources.

◖ Look for assurance scheme logos, for example the Marine Stewardship Council's 'blue tick'.

◖ Be adventurous and try some different fish to help reduce overfishing of the most commonly eaten types.

> **Fish to avoid when pregnant or trying for a baby**
>
> The Food Standards Agency recommends that you should not eat shark, marlin or swordfish if you are pregnant or trying to conceive, owing to the large amounts of mercury now present in these fish.

Get tested
A hair mineral analysis test screens for toxic metals and can also give an indication of your mineral status, including your levels of zinc, selenium and magnesium, which are all vital for fertility. Fertility clinics often offer such tests.

Protect yourself from environmental toxins
There are some simple steps you can take to help minimise your exposure to toxins.

- Buy organic produce wherever possible, but always wash or peel fruit and vegetables prior to eating them.

- Avoid processed foods, smoked food and preserved meats – they all contain nitrous compounds.

- Avoid microwaving food in plastic: cling film is known to leach dangerous chemicals into the food.

- Avoid food and drink in plastic containers or wrapped in plastic.

- Avoid aluminium cookware and aluminium foil.

- Avoid spending too much time walking or exercising along busy roads.

- Stop smoking and avoid smoky environments.

- Refuse dental fillings containing mercury.

- Get outside every day: natural sunlight helps to eliminate toxic metals from the body.

- Avoid using deodorant, hairspray, shower gel and perfume with artificial musks or phthalates.

- Avoid domestic chemical cleaners that contain parabens. Parabens mimic oestrogen and are known to cause hormone disruption and reduce sperm count.

- Avoid using pesticides.

- Limit your use of mobile phones and do not carry your mobile phone in your pocket – this will reduce electromagnetic radiation.

- Avoid using your laptop on your lap.

- Eat foods rich in pectin, like apples and pears, and sulphur foods like garlic and onions, as these are thought to help detoxify heavy metals from your body.

Chapter 5

Testing Times

If you follow the advice in this book regarding diet, exercise, your menstrual cycle, ovulation and stress management, you will give yourself the best possible chance to conceive. It is always worthwhile adopting such an approach first so that you know you have done the best you can to prepare your body for conception. Of course, in some cases, there may be a medical reason why you are still not pregnant, and this chapter looks at some of the common conditions and reasons for infertility and the tests you may need to identify problems.

40. Identify the problem

As mentioned in Chapter 1, fertility problems affect one in eight couples in the UK, although most will go on to conceive within two years.

Getting pregnant isn't always easy: about a quarter of couples take a year or more to conceive. About one in six couples consult an infertility expert, and about one in 80 babies born in the UK are a result of IVF treatment. For many couples, more than one problem makes it difficult for them to conceive. For example, the woman may suffer from endometriosis while her partner may have a low sperm count. Perhaps the most difficult aspect of infertility is when it is unexplained and doctors cannot find a specific medical problem as to why a couple cannot conceive even after thorough investigations.

A few months of trying doesn't necessarily mean you have a fertility problem; it is much more likely that you aren't making love at the right times. Remember: there are only two or three days a month when pregnancy can occur. It's not just about timing: preparing your body for pregnancy is just as important, and fertility experts agree that addressing lifestyle, nutritional and even emotional factors can help and are worthwhile pursuing. It is also worth remembering that fertility declines with age, making it more difficult to conceive as you get older. As fertility testing can be a lengthy process, it is best to make an appointment with your doctor if you think there is a problem and both of you should attend, as fertility problems can affect either men or women or, in some cases, both.

Infertility in the UK

Infertility among couples in the UK is caused by male infertility in 25 per cent of cases and female infertility in 50 per cent of cases, with 25 per cent of those owing to anovulation (the ovaries failing to release an egg during ovulation) and 25 per cent the result of tubal or other problems. Tubal problems are conditions that arise within the Fallopian tubes, such as blockages or damage to the cells. The cause of infertility in 25 per cent of infertile couples is unexplained.

What to expect when you visit your GP

When you visit your doctor he or she will take a medical, sexual and social history from you and your partner. This will include the following:

1. Your ages.

2. The length of time you have been trying to conceive.

3. If you have any other children or have had any miscarriages.

4. Information about your sex life, including any difficulties you may have and how often you have sex.

5. How long it has been since you stopped using contraception and the type of contraception you used.

6. Your medical histories, including if you have had any STIs.

7. Any medication you are taking, including herbal medicines.

8. Your lifestyles, including alcohol, smoking, stress levels, drugs and your weight.

Your GP may then carry out a physical examination and you may be referred to a specialist at an NHS hospital or fertility clinic.

Primary and secondary infertility

There are two types of infertility: primary and secondary. Couples with primary infertility have never been able to conceive, while secondary infertility means difficulty conceiving after already having conceived (and either carried the pregnancy to term or had a miscarriage). Difficulty conceiving with a new partner is not known as secondary infertility.

Causes of infertility in men and women

The factors that cause both male and female infertility include the following:

- Genetic factors, such as a chromosomal abnormality

- Diabetes, thyroid disorders or adrenal disease

- Being either under or overweight

- STIs such as chlamydia

- Smoking

- Exposure to certain chemicals, toxins, metals and solvents

- Stress

Causes of infertility in women

Ovulation disorders

Infertility is often caused by problems with ovulation, which can occur as a result of a number of conditions, including:

- Premature ovarian failure, where a woman's ovaries stop working before she is 40.

- Polycystic ovary syndrome (PCOS), where the ovaries have difficulty producing an egg.

- Thyroid problems, as both an overactive thyroid gland (hypothyroidism) and an underactive thyroid gland can prevent ovulation.

- Chronic long-term conditions such as cancer, which can prevent the ovaries from releasing eggs.

Cushing's syndrome, which is a rare hormonal disease that prevents the ovaries from releasing an egg.

Womb and Fallopian tubes

The Fallopian tubes are the tubes along which the egg travels from the ovary to the womb. The egg is fertilised as it travels down the Fallopian tubes and, when it reaches the womb, it is implanted into the womb's surface, where it continues to grow. If the Fallopian tubes or the womb are damaged or stop working, it may be very difficult to conceive naturally. The following factors may cause this to occur:

Damage to your Fallopian tubes as a result of a previous infection, such as chlamydia, or another condition such as a burst appendix or previous surgery to your Fallopian tubes.

Fibroids, which are non-cancerous growths that can grow on the inside or outside of the womb, in the lining between the uterus and the pelvic cavity.

Endometriosis, which is a condition where small pieces of the womb lining (endometrium) start growing in other places, such as in the Fallopian tubes or the ovaries. These growths form cysts – fluid-filled sacs – or adhesions – sticky areas of tissue – that can distort or block the pelvis, making it difficult for an egg to mature or be released and implanted in the womb.

Pelvic inflammatory disease is an infection of the upper female genital tract, which includes the womb, Fallopian tubes and ovaries. It is usually sexually transmitted and can scar and damage the Fallopian tubes, making it impossible for an egg to travel down into the womb.

Polycystic Ovary Syndrome

PCOS affects millions of women in the UK. Women with PCOS either fail to ovulate or they ovulate infrequently. Polycystic ovary syndrome is one of the most common pelvic disorders for women aged between 15 and 45 years of age: it is thought to affect one in every 15 women in the UK and is considered to be one of the leading causes of female infertility. Women with this disorder have ovaries that contain a large amount of small cysts, which are egg-containing follicles that have not developed properly due to a hormonal imbalance. Women with this condition also tend to have larger ovaries than average.

PCOS can be genetically inherited and, although some women may be more prone to the condition than others, not all will go on to develop PCOS. Factors such as diet and lifestyle are thought to play a role in minimising the chance that PCOS will occur.

Symptoms will vary for each woman; however, the main symptoms include:

- Irregular or lack of menstruation

- Irregular ovulation, or no ovulation at all

- Infertility or recurrent miscarriage

- Acne

- Excess facial or body hair

- Obesity, rapid weight gain

- Depression

PCOS is usually diagnosed by an ultrasound scan and blood tests for hormonal abnormalities and, although it cannot be cured, it can be successfully treated through nutrition, exercise and lifestyle changes. When treating infertility in women suffering from PCOS, Metformin is usually prescribed. The long-term health implications of this condition include diabetes and heart disease.

Pelvic Inflammatory Disease

The most common pelvic disorder is pelvic inflammatory disease, which can affect many women without them even realising it. A serious or longstanding infection like chlamydia can cause scar tissue to build up around a Fallopian tube and prevent the egg from descending. Often, there are few symptoms with this disorder, which is why it makes it so difficult to diagnose initially. An ectopic pregnancy or even a miscarriage can also occur as a result of the disease. It is treated with antibiotics, and surgery is very often required to remove the scar tissue.

Medicines and drugs

The side effects of some medication and drugs may affect your fertility.

- Long-term use of non-steroidal anti-inflammatory drugs, such as aspirin or ibuprofen, can make it more difficult to conceive.

- Chemotherapy, a treatment for cancer, can sometimes cause ovarian failure, which can be permanent.

- Illegal drugs such as cocaine can seriously affect fertility, making ovulation more difficult and affecting the functioning of the Fallopian tubes.

Age

As we have already seen, infertility is linked to age; it begins to decline during a woman's mid-30s.

The hormonal link

PCOS, fibroids and endometriosis are known to be linked to excess oestrogen production and the overproduction of prostaglandins – hormones that play an important role in the fertilisation and implantation of the embryo.

Physical examination

Your doctor may weigh you when carrying out a physical examination to see if you have a healthy BMI, as well as examining your pelvic area to check for vaginal infection or tenderness which could indicate endometriosis or pelvic inflammatory disease.

41. Learn about fertility tests for men and women

There are different types of fertility tests for men and women. Generally, the tests for women are more complicated than those for men, as they are based on hormone levels during the monthly cycle, which are likely to fluctuate.

Tests for female infertility

Progesterone test

A blood test is taken to determine if you are ovulating. The progesterone test will be taken seven days before you expect your period to start, so it is important you know your cycle, as this only works if you have a regular 28-day cycle. You must inform your

GP if this is not the case so they can work out when to take your blood, otherwise you are likely to get the wrong information. The progesterone test is also known as the 21-day test.

Hormone tests

If your periods are irregular, your follicle-stimulating hormone and luteinising hormone levels may be tested through a routine blood test. From this it may be possible for you to be given an indication of the quality of your eggs and of your ovarian reserve; your store of eggs decreases as you age. Your prolactin hormone level may also be tested if you have any symptoms of an ovulation disorder such as PCOS.

Thyroid function test

Between approximately 1.3 per cent and 5.1 per cent of infertile women have an abnormal thyroid. If you have any symptoms of a thyroid abnormality (including weight loss or weight gain), your thyroid may be tested to see if it is working properly.

Chlamydia test

This STI will affect fertility and your GP will use a swab, similar to a cotton bud but smaller and more rounded, to collect some cells from your cervix. Antibiotics will be prescribed if you are suffering from chlamydia.

Sexually transmitted infections

STIs such as chlamydia and gonorrhoea are on the increase and affect fertility. Very often, these infections can go undiagnosed owing to a lack of symptoms. Your GP or consultant will often test for these infections when you seek medical help for infertility.

Chlamydia is very prevalent among under-25s who have been sexually active; the National Chlamydia Screening Programme (www.

chlamydiascreening.nhs.uk) offers free chlamydia testing to men and women in this age group. DIY chlamydia tests are also available from pharmacies and colleges.

Genito-urinary infections

Any inflammation or infection of the genito-urinary (GU) system can affect your fertility. Research found that 69 per cent of patients at an infertility clinic in the UK suffered from GU infections. In men, GU infections may cause damaged sperm and blocked ducts in the testes, while in women these infections can lead to pelvic inflammatory disease.

Other infections

There are several other infections that can seriously affect both men and women's fertility. They include:

Cytomegalovirus, which is caused by the herpes virus and can reduce a man's sperm count.

Mycoplasmas, which are small organisms found in everyone but which are present in greater numbers in those experiencing fertility problems. They are not tested for on the NHS, so you would have to go for private screening. It is worthwhile screening for these if you have had a miscarriage.

Genital herpes, which is a sexually transmitted virus and can increase the risk of miscarriage.

The next series of tests looks for blockages in the Fallopian tubes, as these may prevent the sperm from travelling to the egg, or the descent of the egg. These tests are usually carried out during the first half of your menstrual cycle. They include:

⬛ A hysterosalpingography, which is a type of X-ray procedure where a special dye is injected through your cervix to check the inside of your womb (uterus) for any abnormalities and to look for blockages or abnormalities such as scar tissue or tumours in your Fallopian tubes. If there are any blockages, your specialist may recommend a laparoscopy, where a narrow instrument with a telescopic lens is inserted through a small incision just below the navel to see the womb, Fallopian tubes and ovaries. This will require a general anaesthetic and will allow the specialist to look for anything unusual, such as endometriosis or fibroids.

⬛ A hysteroscopy, which can sometimes be carried out at the same time as a laparoscopy. This test involves a slim tube-like telescopic camera being passed through the vagina and cervix to look inside your womb.

⬛ A hysterosalpingo-contrast sonography, which is a type of ultrasound scan that is used instead of X-rays to check your Fallopian tubes. A small amount of fluid will be injected into your womb through a tube put into your cervix and high-frequency sound waves will be used to create an image of your womb and Fallopian tubes to highlight any abnormalities.

Tests for male infertility

Male infertility is the reason for infertility in nearly one third of couples experiencing problems conceiving. Generally, male infertility can be grouped into four major categories: abnormal sperm, atypical hormone production, damage to the testes, and genetic problems. The most common cause is a problem with sperm: approximately 10–15 per cent of men have sperm problems. Approximately 30 per cent of male infertility problems are never identified.

Physical examination

Your GP will usually start with a physical examination, where he will check the testicles for any abnormalities, including varicocele, a condition similar to varicose veins in the testicles, or lumps. Not all men with this condition suffer infertility problems; however, the condition does result in poor blood flow and is generally thought to be responsible for sperm damage. The doctor will also check the shape and structure of the penis for any abnormalities.

Sperm and semen analysis

A semen analysis is non-invasive, although ejaculation has to be avoided for two to four days before the sample is given. Testing will determine sperm count, mobility and motility issues or abnormal sperm. A lack viable or motile of sperm in the semen in the sample is known as azoospermia, which can result from a blockage in the tubes. It can be corrected through surgery.

Chlamydia test

Just as for women, the GP may test for chlamydia with a urine sample. If the test is positive, antibiotics will be prescribed.

Hormone tests

A blood test will indicate levels of the key sex hormones FSH, LH and testosterone.

Other tests

Ultrasound scanning, biopsy and genetic screening may also be offered, depending on the results of the sperm and semen test.

42. Understand your fertility problems

Once you have both been tested and have some idea as to what may be the underlying cause of infertility, you will be able to think about your next steps. You should try to understand as much as possible about your diagnosis so that you can both consider the implications of trying for a baby. Zita West believes that combining conventional and complementary therapies along with good nutrition and lifestyle changes, if necessary, will give you the best chance to improve your condition and increase your fertility.

Getting support

If you have always suspected that you have fertility problems, it will probably come as some sort of relief to discover the outcome of the tests. However, if you had no idea, receiving news that you may have a problem conceiving can be difficult; you may need to find support from your partner, family and others to help you at this time. There are several support groups that you can call on (see the Directory) and your GP will also be able to help and may refer you to a counsellor.

43. Take natural steps to improve your fertility

Although PCOS, fibroids and endometriosis are very different conditions, they can all be triggered by hormone imbalances, nutritional deficiencies and stress. Eating a healthy diet, watching your weight and learning to relax will significantly improve these conditions and can improve your fertility. Try some of these suggestions:

Cut back on saturated fat: not only does it overstimulate the production of oestrogen, which is linked to all three conditions, it also produces hormones called prostaglandins, which make endometriosis cramps more painful.

Reduce sugar, as it increases fat and oestrogen production.

Reduce or eliminate caffeine, as it rids the body of vital nutrients, including vitamins and minerals.

Increase your fibre intake, as this helps to reduce oestrogen levels.

Eliminate alcohol, as it can have a direct affect upon the liver. If this major organ cannot function properly, harmful toxins build up and adversely affect general health.

Exercise to reduce stress.

Ensure an adequate intake of essential fatty acids found in fish, vegetables oils, nuts and seeds.

Chapter 6

Medical Treatment and Assisted Conception

By now, if you have followed the advice in this book regarding diet, exercise and stress management you will have prepared your body for the opportunity to conceive. As we have seen, however, sometimes lifestyle changes are not enough for natural conception, and after seeking medical help and having tests to determine the cause (or causes) of infertility you may be considering the use of assisted reproductive technology to help you conceive. You can of course improve your chances of successful treatment through an appropriate diet and lifestyle changes.

According to the British Fertility Society one in six couples will seek infertility treatment. Perhaps the most well known treatment is *in vitro* fertilisation (IVF), but there are a number of other options including fertility drugs, surgery and a range of assisted reproduction technologies.

This chapter gives you an overview of some of the treatments commonly used to assist conception, as well as discussing the psychological effects of being unable to conceive and give birth to a child.

Eligibility for treatment

Fertility treatment that is funded by the NHS is available across the UK. In some areas waiting lists for fertility treatment are long and the criteria you need to meet to be eligible for treatment can vary from area to area. Your doctor is the best person to advise you on this and if you are referred for treatment the costs will be covered by the NHS. All patients have the right to be referred to a NHS clinic for an initial investigation.

Understanding your treatment

No medical treatment is entirely free from complications and risk, and infertility treatment is no exception. However, most women go through IVF and assisted conception treatment without serious problems. Should you discover that your treatment produces adverse side effects you should contact your specialist immediately for advice.

Private treatment

Many couples experiencing fertility problems may consider private treatment which can be very expensive and, as with any other treatment, there is no guarantee that it will be successful. If you do decide to choose a private clinic then make sure the clinic is licensed by the Human Fertilisation and Embryology Authority (HFEA), which is a government organisation that regulates and inspects all UK clinics that provide fertility treatment, including the storage of eggs, sperm and embryos. Also ask for a personalised treatment plan so that you have some idea of the costs you may experience.

44. Know your fertility treatment options

Your treatment will very much depend upon your type of fertility problem and what is available from your primary care trust (PCT). Your GP will be able to advise you of this.

Medicines to assist fertility

Usually these are given to women, but occasionally they may also be prescribed for men.

Ovulation induction (OI) is a method of regulating the menstrual cycle so ovulation occurs. It is usually recommended for women whose periods are irregular and who do not ovulate regularly or cannot ovulate at all, or if they have polycystic ovary syndrome (PCOS) or a luteal phase defect where insufficient amounts of progesterone are produced.

The drug used in ovulation induction is clomiphene citrate, better known as clomifene or clomid. It increases the levels of two reproduction hormones, FSH and LH, which in turn causes stimulation of the ovaries which release an egg. Available in tablet form, it is administered for up to six cycles, although it takes at least two cycles before ovulation occurs, after which, if it has not proved successful, your doctor or consultant may begin to discuss other options. Clomifene may be given before undergoing IVF to encourage the production of eggs for the procedure. Men with certain hormonal imbalances linked to a low sperm count, or poor sperm motility or quality, may also be given clomifene.

Tamoxifen

Commonly used as a hormonal therapy that lowers the risk of recurrence in women with hormone-receptor-positive breast cancer, tamoxifen increases ovulation and is given in higher doses when treating fertility problems. It is considered to be an alternative to clomifene, especially if you are unable to take the latter.

Metaformin

Metaformin is an insulin-sensitising drug and usually prescribed to treat diabetes. It is also given to women with polycystic ovary syndrome (PCOS) and ovulation problems, or for those who have a body mass index (BMI) of 25 and over. It may be prescribed if clomifene has not worked, but can also be used at the same time.

Gonadotrophins

Gonadotrophin-releasing hormone agonists stimulate the release of natural sex hormones from the brain. They may be prescribed if you have failed to respond to clomifene, or have not become pregnant but have ovulated after using clomifene, have polycystic ovary syndrome, or are about to embark on assisted conception treatment. Gonadotrophins directly affect the ovaries and stimulate follicle development, unlike clomifene, which stimulates the pituitary gland. There are several types of gonadotrophins: human menopausal gonadotrophins (hMG) consist of FSH and LH, while recombinant or urofollitropin Gonadotrophins are purely from FSHs. You will be given one or the other in a course of injections for 7–12 days to stimulate the ovaries to produce several eggs. After this, another injection of human chorionic gonadotrophin (hCG) is given to encourage the ovaries to release mature eggs into the Fallopian tubes.

Gonadotrophins can also be given to men with a low sperm count. These drugs go under the following brand names:

- Pergonal, Humegon, Repronex (containing LH and FSH)
- Metrodin, Fertinex, Follistim, Gonal F (containing FSH)
- Perganyl (containing hCG)

The success rate of fertility drugs

Around 70 per cent of women using drugs to stimulate ovulation will be successful and will ovulate within the first three months of treatment. Of those who ovulate, 15–50 per cent will become pregnant. Very few pregnancies occur after six months of taking clomifene.

Side effects

As with all drugs there are often side effects with fertility drugs; minor side effects may include mood swings, nausea, stomach pain, mild ovarian swelling, breast tenderness, insomnia, vomiting, blurred vision, fatigue, headaches, irritability, depression, weight gain and, in much rarer cases, ovarian cysts.

Ultrasound scans are needed to check the number and development of follicles in the ovaries. Clomifene requires regular monitoring.

Ovarian hyperstimulation syndrome (OHSS), where the ovaries swell to several times their normal size due to excessive egg production, can sometimes occur and is a potentially fatal condition. Fertility drugs can result in the production of more than one egg being released, increasing the chances of multiple pregnancy.

Surgical Procedures

There is a variety of surgical procedures that are used for treating infertility. Your consultant will determine your treatment depending upon the problem (or problems) that you and your partner may be experiencing. Some common conditions and the surgery used to correct them are listed below:

Fallopian tube surgery

If the Fallopian tubes have become blocked or are scarred from pelvic inflammatory disorder (PID) then surgery to repair the tubes and clear the scar tissue may be required.

Laparoscopic surgery

A cut is made in the abdomen so a small microscope (laparoscope) can be passed through the incision to look at the internal organs. This treatment is very good for determining if a woman has endometriosis (when parts of the womb grow outside of the womb), as well as to remove cysts and fibroids.

Surgery to correct an epididymal blockage

This procedure is for men, and is performed on the epididymis, a coil-like structure in the testicles, which stores and transports sperm. If the epididymis becomes blocked it prevents sperm from being ejaculated normally. Surgery can correct the blockage and sperm is once again able to flow properly.

Assisted conception

There are several different techniques used to carry out artificial insemination or assisted conception, which are available on the NHS. They include the following:

Intrauterine insemination (IUI)

IUI is the most widely used technique on the NHS and has a good success record. Your partner will have to provide a sperm sample, which is then washed and filtered so the best quality sperm can be inserted into your womb through a fine plastic tube (a catheter) at a time that coincides with ovulation. You may also be offered a low dose of ovary-stimulating hormones at the same time in order to maximise the chances of conception. This treatment tends to be used when infertility cannot be explained, if you have mild endometriosis, or if your partner has a low sperm count, decreased sperm motility, is impotent or ejaculates too quickly. The success rate for IUI is around 15 per cent for each cycle of treatment for women under 35, providing the Fallopian tubes and the sperm are both healthy.

IUI can also be used with a donor's sperm – donor insemination (DI) – if your partner is unable to provide sperm or if you do not have a male partner.

If IUI is unsuccessful you may then wish to discuss IVF treatment with your consultant.

The National Institute for Health and Clinical Excellence (NICE) recommends that couples should be offered up to six cycles of IUI, which are granted if:

1. Your partner's sperm count is abnormal.

2. You have minimal to mild endometriosis.

3. As a couple you have unexplained infertility problems.

However, bear in mind that availability from your PCT and the criteria you may need to meet can vary in every area and waiting lists for treatment can be very long. IUI is also available at private fertility clinics but will come at considerable cost.

In vitro fertilisation (IVF)

IVF is better known as the 'test tube' method of conceiving, in which fertilisation takes place outside of the body. A drug to suppress the natural menstrual cycle is given and then a fertility drug is administered to encourage the ovaries to produce more eggs than usual. The eggs are then removed from the ovaries and fertilised with sperm in a laboratory dish. Once fertilised the eggs become known as embryos and are put back into the woman's body.

For women under the age of 40, one or two embryos can be transferred; for women over 40 a maximum of three embryos can be put back. There are several different methods used for this treatment, but be aware that not all of them are available on the NHS. They include blastocyst transfer, where the embryos are left to mature for five to six days and then transferred, or assisted hatching, when the shell of the egg is made thinner or a hole made in the shell to help the embryo hatch.

A clinic may recommend IVF if you have been diagnosed with unexplained infertility, if your Fallopian tubes are blocked or if you have been unsuccessful with IUI treatment.

NICE recommends that up to three cycles of IVF should be offered to couples if you fulfill the following criteria:

1. You are 23–39 years of age at the time of treatment.

2. The cause of your infertility problems has been identified.

3. You have had infertility problems for at least three years.

The NHS aims to provide at least one funded cycle of IVF treatment for couples that meet these criteria. NICE recommends that it is appropriate to fund IVF treatment when the chances of success are more than 10 per cent. Priority is given to couples that do not already have a child living with them. The success rate for IVF is 29 per cent for women who are under 35 years of age. The success rate decreases as a woman's age increases.

In vitro maturation (IVM)

In IVM eggs are removed from the ovaries and collected while they are still immature. They are then matured in the laboratory before being fertilised. This form of assisted conception may be recommended if you are susceptible to developing OHSS (ovarian hyperstimulation syndrome) due to fertility drugs, if you have PCOS (polycystic ovary syndrome), or if infertility has been identified as being a male factor only. It is similar to IVF, in that the eggs are fertilised with your partner's sperm in the laboratory and placed back into the womb, but different in that you do not need to take as many drugs as IVF due to the immaturity of the eggs being collected. The success rate of IVM is similar to IVF, though IVM is a relatively new treatment.

Other assisted conception techniques available

Donor insemination (DI)
It is possible to utilise sperm from a donor who will have been screened for genetic diseases and sexually transmitted diseases. In the majority of cases sperm donation is usually anonymous and IUI is used. You may also be able to receive eggs from a donor if your own eggs are not suitable.

Genetic testing
Pre-implantation genetic testing involves testing embryos created through IVF or ICSI treatment to detect certain inherited genetic conditions or abnormalities and helps to prevent affected embryos being transferred to the womb.

Gamete intra-Fallopian transfer (GIFT)
Although eggs are taken from the ovaries, the healthiest are selected and placed together with sperm in your Fallopian tubes, so fertilisation occurs within the body. However, this technique is not available through the NHS.

Treatments for male infertility
The same fertility drugs that stimulate ovulation also stimulate sperm production and are prescribed where there are problems with sperm count.

Unfortunately, the fertility drugs do not work as effectively for men; success rates are about a third of that of women and the drugs are only used for men with a specific hormone imbalance. The most likely drugs to be prescribed for men include clomifene and human menopausal gonadotrophin (hMG), used with human chorionic gonadotrophin (hCG). These fertility drugs are used to treat primary hypogonadotrophic hypogonadism, a testosterone deficiency in the pituitary gland that prevents the testicles from receiving the signal to make sperm. Clomifene is given in tablet form, whilst hCG is injected two to three times a week, sometimes with hMG.

Intra-cytoplasmic sperm injection (ICSI)

This is a technique used for male infertility or for patients who have been unsuccessful with IVF treatment. It is very similar to IVF, however a single sperm is injected into a single egg in the laboratory. The fertilised egg is then transferred to the womb.

Counselling

It has long been recognised that infertility is very traumatic and that fertility treatment for couples can produce stress and trauma. In 1990 Parliament decided that all assisted clinics must provide a counselling service for their patients. The emotional impact of infertility may affect you before, during and even after treatment, which is why you should consider this service where it is available to you. The British Infertility Counselling Association (BICA), whose details are in the Directory section of this book, offer a service specifically for couples undertaking fertility treatment and will find a counsellor in your local area if you do not wish to use the clinic's counsellor or want additional support.

The aim of counselling is to help you understand exactly what the treatment will involve and how it may affect you and your partner. Very often one or both of you may feel depressed or anxious at times when dealing with your infertility, so having someone to share these feelings and emotions with in a non-judgmental, safe environment may prove very useful. Fertility treatments can challenge most relationships and taking care of yourself at this time is especially important.

The Infertility Network UK

This national charity offers practical and emotional support to all those suffering from infertility.
www.infertilitynetworkuk.com.

Chapter 7

Complementary Therapies

Complementary therapies, also known as alternative, natural or holistic therapies, approach health problems and conditions by focusing on the individual as a whole, as opposed to conventional treatment which is symptom-led. Complementary therapists view illness as a sign that mental and physical health has been disrupted, leading to a state of imbalance. Zita West, a fertility expert and midwife to the actress Kate Winslet, believes complementary therapies can encourage conception by helping to bring the body back into balance, although they may not necessarily be a cure for infertility. Of course, many will argue that the benefits experienced by complementary therapies are due to a placebo effect, whereby treatment brings about an improvement simply because the person using it expects it to, rather than because it is having any real effect. However, it can be argued that complementary therapies such as massage, reflexology and acupuncture have been used for centuries to treat various ailments and illness.

This chapter offers a brief overview of the complementary therapies that may aid fertility and includes acupuncture, homeopathy, reflexology, aromatherapy, Bach flower remedies, yoga and qigong.

45. Apply acupuncture

A traditional Chinese medicinal therapy that has been practised for over 2,000 years, acupuncture is one of the most popular alternative treatments for infertility and is often used alongside conventional fertility treatments like IVF and IUI in fertility clinics. Midwife Zita West routinely uses acupuncture on her patients at her fertility clinic in London.

Acupuncture works by restoring the energy flow through the body. It is based on the idea that we all have a life energy, or *qi*, which flows along invisible channels – meridians – in the body, and passes through acupoints, or acupuncture points located along the meridians, which are like pathways in the body. When one of these pathways becomes blocked, disease, illness or pain occurs. The meridians associated with the reproductive system include the kidneys, spleen and liver and are found on one of 12 meridian lines called the 'conception meridian'. Sterilised needles are placed at these points in order to restore the blood flow and *qi*.

Research has shown that acupuncture can help relieve some of the symptoms of conditions such as painful periods, menstrual cycle irregularities, absence of periods, hormonal imbalance and fibroids, which may compromise fertility, whilst it is widely accepted that acupuncture enhances relaxation, lowers stress levels and increases endorphins ('feel-good' hormones) and encephalins (pain-relieving hormones).

Certain studies have shown that women receiving both IVF and acupuncture together are more likely to conceive than women having IVF treatment alone. Acupuncture is thought to help improve male fertility problems; a German study found that male patients receiving ten sessions of acupuncture all showed a significant improvement in sperm quality.

As with most complementary therapies, it is worthwhile finding a qualified acupuncture practitioner who specialises in treating those with fertility problems.

46. Get help with homeopathy

Homeopathy is a system of medicine that works on the basis of 'like cures like' – meaning, a substance that would cause symptoms in a healthy person is used to cure those same symptoms in illness. For example, a person suffering from insomnia may be given coffee (which can cause sleeplessness) as a remedy, using a highly diluted substance given mainly in tablet form, although they can also be prescribed in tincture or powder form. Homeopaths claim that the more diluted the remedy is the higher its potency and the lower its potential side effects. Homeopathy treats the individual, so all remedies are tailor-made and the theory is that homeopathic remedies – which come from natural substances found in animals, minerals or plants – encourage self-healing, as they work in a similar way to vaccines, stimulating the body's defences against the disease or problem.

Homeopathy is not without its sceptics, and although evidence to support homeopathy exists many critics argue that it is inconclusive. For those who remain convinced, homeopathy is considered to improve overall reproductive health and can be used to treat both female and male fertility problems. According to Dr Bob Leckridge, a homeopath at the Glasgow Homeopathic Hospital, prescribing women with fertility problems the same hormone that is causing the problem can aid fertility. Folliculinum, for example, is prescribed for women who are not ovulating properly and is an extract of ovarian follicle, thought to help stimulate the reproductive system.

In a randomised, placebo-controlled double-blind study conducted in Germany more than half the women with fertility problems experienced improved ovulation or pregnancy after taking a homeopathic remedy.

It is best to consult a qualified homeopath who will prescribe a personal remedy dependent upon your symptoms. You can buy homeopathic remedies over the counter at most pharmacies, such as Boots. To self-prescribe, simply choose the remedy that most closely resembles your symptoms and follow the dosage on the product.

The following homeopathic remedies are suitable for helping with female infertility:

- Sepia 6c: useful if you suffer from irregular or absent ovulation.

- Folliculinum: for irregular ovulation.

- Aurum: used when low sex drive and depression contribute towards infertility.

- Phosphorus: used when anxiety and stress are contributing to female infertility.

- Sabina 6c: recommended for women who have experienced recurrent miscarriage.

The following homeopathic remedies are recommended for male infertility:

- Sepia 6c: useful for men experiencing low libido and sex drive.

- Medorrhinum: considered useful for men experiencing impotence.

47. Find relief in reflexology

Reflexology is based on the principle that certain points on the feet are linked to various organs and systems of the body, including the ovaries and Fallopian tubes. When these points – known as 'reflexes' and linked via vertical zones along which energy flows – are blocked, illness occurs. Stimulation of the reflexes by using the fingers and thumbs is thought to bring about physiological changes, which remove these blockages and encourage the body to self-heal.

Reflexology aids relaxation and reduces stress levels. It is thought to help fertility by boosting blood circulation, balancing hormones and regulating the menstrual cycle, and is considered beneficial for women suffering from PCOS (polycystic ovary syndrome) and endometriosis. Reflexology is thought to benefit men with a low sperm count or low sperm motility.

DIY reflexology

If you wish to apply reflexology yourself then use your thumbs or two forefingers and massage the corresponding area on either your foot or hand in a circular motion, or use the press and release technique detailed below. Very often you will know if you have the right area, as it will be painful when you apply your pressure.

Boost your fertility

Apply firm pressure to the middle of your big toe. This stimulates the ovaries and triggers the release of the hormone prostaglandin.

Activate your ovary reflexes

Using the middle finger of one hand, apply pressure to the area just in front of your wrist bone, below your little finger on the other hand. Hold for a few seconds, release and repeat three times.

Alleviate stress

Apply pressure directly under the ball of your foot under the big toe. It is thought this technique soothes the adrenal glands, which are often stressed from everyday life. The adrenal glands help to regulate your hormones. Another area that stimulates the adrenal glands is found on the hands. Using the thumb of one hand apply a firm pressure to the point between the thumb and forefinger, a couple of centimeters into your palm, on your other hand. Hold for a few seconds, release and repeat three times on each palm.

48. Use aroma power

Aromatherapy is the use of essential oils; highly concentrated plant substances extracted from roots, seeds, barks and leaves that can be used in massage, baths, inhalers and compresses to promote physical and psychological well-being. It is thought the scent released from the essential oils when they are inhaled affects the hypothalamus, the part of the brain that regulates the glands and hormones, altering mood and lowering stress levels. The oils are absorbed into the bloodstream via the skin and transported around the body to the organs and glands that benefit from their healing effects.

Aromatherapy has, like so many complementary therapies, been used for over a thousand years and well-tested combinations of essential oils have been used to stimulate the central nervous system, whilst relieving tension and stress.

Although there is no direct evidence to show aromatherapy will help you conceive, many aromatherapists believe it has a direct beneficial affect upon fertility and clinical trials have found essential oils can cause changes to the pituitary gland, affect hormone production and stimulate the brain. A practising aromatherapist may recommend oils such as rose, lavender, chamomile and jasmine as these are known to help regulate the menstrual cycle and encourage hormone balance. However, aromatherapy is also beneficial for relieving tension, anxiety and stress, which in itself is likely to have a very positive effect on fertility.

Essential oils can be bought over the counter at most high street chemists or pharmacies. Tisserand Aromatherapy and Natural by Nature Oils offer a wide range of good quality essential oils – contact details are in the Useful Products section. Should you decide to try aromatherapy yourself, the recommended concentration of essential oils is no more than 2.5 per cent for adults. One teaspoon (5 ml) of carrier oil equals 100 drops. As a rough guide, add two drops of essential oil per 5 ml of carrier oil. You can use good quality – ideally organic – olive, sunflower or sesame oils if you have them in your kitchen cupboard.

Hormone-balancing oils
Fennel, geranium, and chamomile along with clary sage and rose are all useful for balancing hormones. Clary sage is golden yellow oil with a deep, earthy smell and is thought to be very beneficial when applied over the reproductive organs to help balance oestrogen levels. It is also an aphrodisiac, as is rose, with its sweet-smelling, uplifting scent. Rose is thought to help tone and cleanse the uterus; however, when used for men it is thought to increase sperm count. Ideally, get your partner to take a warm (not hot) bath with several drops of rose oil added to improve sperm levels.

Stress relievers
Clary sage, lavender, bergamot, patchouli, chamomile, jasmine, rose, ylang-ylang and frankincense are all great stress relievers and help to restore energy. For the quickest and easiest way to experience the healing effects, either inhale the oil's aroma by putting two to three

drops of oil on a tissue or your pillow before you sleep and breathe deeply, or diffuse the oils into the air by mixing with two to three drops of water into an oil burner and filling the room with scent.

Enjoy a lavender and rose bath

For a relaxing bath try adding lavender and rose oil, adding eight drops of each under the running water. If you feel anxious as well then add geranium, but reduce the drops of each oil from eight to five.

Important: fennel oil is not recommended for anyone with epilepsy.

Essential oils should not be applied directly to the skin but should be diluted in carrier oil such as almond, avocado, wheatgerm or grapeseed to prevent skin irritation.

Flower power!

Flower essences have been used for centuries; however, it was Edward Bach, a doctor, bacteriologist and homeopath, who first developed their use in the twentieth century. The remedies, developed after Bach identified 38 basic negative states of mind and devised a remedy for each, are thought to counteract negative emotions including depression and anxiety, relieving stress and emotional imbalances such as fear, despair and uncertainty. These emotions can affect the body's ability to reach optimum health, as experiencing prolonged negative emotions at a psychological level can negatively affect the body at a physical level.

Although there is only anecdotal evidence regarding their effectiveness, many people find them useful and flower essences are available over the counter in pharmacies. They come in handy 10 ml or 20 ml bottles, which can be discreetly carried in your handbag or briefcase. They are completely natural and can be used with any conventional medicine.

Gentian is useful for feelings of despondency and discouragement, white chestnut for constant worrying thoughts and agrimony if you are experiencing inner anguish. The Bach Rescue Remedy is made up of five individual flower essences and designed to help you cope in times of acute stress, which may be very useful, for example, if you are going through IVF treatment. For further details visit www.bachfloweressences.co.uk or www.nelsonsnaturalworld.com.

49. Say 'yes' to yoga

Although there are many different forms of yoga, one of the best for increasing fertility is considered to be hatha yoga. Ideally, refrain from practising Bikram or hot yoga and ashtanga yoga, as these are not beneficial for fertility.

There are thought to be six yoga poses that help to increase fertility. Try to practise them at least three times a week.

1. Lotus Pose – Sit on the floor or on a mat with your legs crossed and your back very straight. Rest the back of your hands on your knees. If you are having trouble keeping your back straight then fold up a blanket and place it under your bottom. Breathe in and out gently and relax. Hold the pose for at least 30 seconds, and up to several minutes.

2. Legs up the wall – lie on your back with your legs resting up on the wall in front of you. Your head, shoulders and arms should be resting on the floor. Allow the knees to relax as you breathe gently and slowly. Hold the pose for a few minutes then gently lower your knees to your chest and over to one side. Do not practise this pose if you are menstruating.

3. Butterfly Pose – Sit on the floor or your mat with your back straight and put the soles of your feet together. Pull your feet gently in towards your body with your hands and breathe deeply. Hold the pose for at least 30 seconds.

4. Child's Pose – This is a very relaxing pose. Kneel on the floor or on your mat and, keeping your bottom on your heels, slide your arms and chest forwards towards the ground, out in front of you. Try and rest your forehead on the floor. Breathe in and out gently and hold the pose for several minutes.

5. Pelvic Tilt Pose – This pose helps to stimulate blood flow through the pelvic region. Lie on your back on the floor or on your mat and bend your knees, keeping your feet flat on the floor. Rest your arms down by your sides. Breathe in and, as you breathe out, lift your pelvis and push it towards the ceiling. Take three slow long breaths and then gradually relax your spine back down to the floor.

6. Supported Bridge Pose – This is similar to the pelvic tilt pose and has similar benefits. Lie on your back with your knees bent and your arms resting by your sides. Bring your feet in as close to your bottom as you can, then, taking two deep breaths, raise your pelvis whilst keeping your inner thighs and feet close together. Bring your hands together underneath your back. Hold the pose for one minute, breathing deeply and slowly.

50. Breathe it away

Qigong is the Mandarin Chinese term used to describe – among various other techniques – the art of controlled breathing. This form of self-healing therapy implies that through practice the individual is able to take control of *qi*, a form of life energy. Qigong requires you to learn to breath using the entire lung – normally most of us take shallow breaths, using only the top section of the lungs. When more oxygen is circulated around the body and delivered to the vital organs it brings with it a feeling of relaxation, helps to eliminate and control stress and cultivates healthy energy.

A simple deep-breathing exercise such as the one below may help you to feel more relaxed. It is also thought to improve kidney function and make the blood in the uterus more abundant, encouraging fertility.

You can practise this technique lying or sitting down.

1. Close your eyes and try to relax your mind.

2. Place the tip of your tongue on the roof of your mouth just behind the top of your front teeth.

3. Breathe deeply in through your nose and concentrate on taking the breath down through the midline of your body to your abdomen.

4. Focusing on your lower abdomen, gently contract your pelvic floor muscles, as if stopping yourself from urinating.

5. Then relax and exhale the breath fully from your abdomen, feeling the breath travelling up through the midline of your body and out through your nose and mouth.

Repeat this process several times a day or whenever you feel anxious or stressed.

Remember: help is at hand

It can be very difficult to cope when you are not able to get pregnant. Many couples choose treatment options to try and become pregnant, some seek egg or sperm donors, while others look at the possibility of adoption; either way, it is very important to deal with the feelings surrounding infertility before making important decisions.

Make sure that whichever path you choose you do so with the best support around you; from your doctor to your consultant, your family and friends, to support groups with others who are experiencing the same thing. However, be sure that it is your decision and that you weren't talked into it. A list of support groups is in the Directory at the back of this book.

Support is vital to help you and your partner, especially if difficulties should arise between you. Make sure you understand your fertility problem and all of your options, as it's important to get the facts so you can deal with the myths. Realise that men and women deal with infertility differently; according to studies men are thought to be about five years behind their partners emotionally in dealing with their infertility problems, and the expectation from others on women to have children is often greater.

Even if you do get pregnant through fertility treatment, you may still feel the grief of not having been able to have a child naturally and may benefit from seeking help. Of course, some couples choose to be child-free; it gives them the opportunity to turn their situation into a positive experience and allows them to move forward with their decision.

Recipes

This section contains recipes based on some of the dietary recommendations outlined in this book.

Relaxation Smoothie (serves 1)

This smoothie is rich in antioxidants, vitamins A, C and E and is beneficial for your digestive system.

Ingredients

½ chopped mango
1 chopped banana
150 ml apple juice

Method

Blend all the ingredients together and serve.

Vitality Smoothie (serves 1)

This smoothie is high in nutrients including Vitamin E, protein, calcium, zinc, magnesium and B vitamins, all vital for helping to regulate hormones. The high vitamin E content makes it ideal for aiding conception and boosting energy for both males and females.

Ingredients

150 ml low fat yoghurt
250 ml skimmed cows' or goats' milk
1 sliced banana
2 tablespoons natural/rolled oats
2 tablespoons wheatgerm
1 teaspoon runny honey

Method

Place the banana, honey, wheatgerm, low fat yoghurt and rolled oats into a blender for 30 seconds. Add the milk and blend again to milkshake consistency. Serve.

Chicken and Bean Salad (serves 4)

The chicken, kidney beans and chickpeas provide B vitamins, magnesium, folate and zinc. The beans have a stabilising effect on the menstrual cycle, help to reduce PMS symptoms and lower the risk of fibroids, whilst the peppers are high in antioxidants.

Ingredients

110 g cooked chicken breast (no skin)
110 g soaked and cooked kidney beans
110 g soaked and cooked chickpeas
50 g sliced red pepper
50 g sliced leeks
50 g sliced mushrooms
1–2 tablespoons lemon juice
1 tablespoon runny honey
Pinch paprika
Pinch cayenne pepper

Method

Shred the chicken breast into a large bowl and mix with kidney beans, chickpeas, pepper, leeks and mushrooms. Add the honey and the lemon juice, cayenne pepper and paprika. Season with salt and pepper and serve.

Watercress Soup (serves 4)

Watercress not only provides B vitamins but also a range of minerals including calcium, potassium, iron, sodium, magnesium and zinc. It is also thought to be helpful for menstruation problems and provides energy due to the high content of B vitamins. The brown rice has a low GI and is also full of B vitamins and provides essential fibre.

Ingredients

1 onion
2 ½ cups watercress
2 ½ cups vegetable stock
1 ¼ cups low fat milk
¾ cup low fat yoghurt
2 tablespoons brown rice

Method

Chop and fry the onion until soft in a saucepan; add the rice, watercress and stock and simmer until the rice is tender, then purée. Stir in the milk and yoghurt and reheat gently. Season to taste. Serve with wholegrain or rye bread.

Baked Trout with Tarragon (serves 2)

The trout is an oily fish and therefore high in polyunsaturated fats: omega-3 and omega-6 – essential fatty acids. These fatty acids cannot be manufactured by the body and have to be found in the foods you eat. They are thought to play an important role in fertility by regulating hormones and may improve sperm motility. They are also high in vitamins, including A, D, E and K, as well as minerals including selenium, zinc, magnesium and phosphorous.

Ingredients

2 x 350–450 g rainbow trout cleaned and gutted
2 sprigs tarragon
Lemon slices to garnish
Olive oil

Method

Coat the insides of the fish with a little olive oil to prevent it from drying out. Place a sprig of tarragon and some lemon slices inside the cavity of the fish. Season lightly with salt and pepper and place in the preheated oven at gas mark 5 (190°C/375°F) for 20–25 minutes. The fish should be fork tender. Serve with steamed vegetables or salad.

Lentil Pilaf with Mushrooms and Spinach (serves 4)

Lentils are packed with protein and rich in fibre, iron, potassium and B vitamins along with the essential amino acids, lysine and isoleucine.

Ingredients

1 onion
2 chopped garlic cloves
Extra virgin olive oil
½ cup lentils
½ cup brown rice
½ cup wild rice
2 ½ cups vegetable stock
1 tablespoon chopped fresh thyme

Method

Sauté the onion and garlic in the oil until soft then add the lentils, rice and stock and bring to the boil. Simmer gently until the stock has reduced and then add the chopped thyme and serve with spinach and salad leaves.

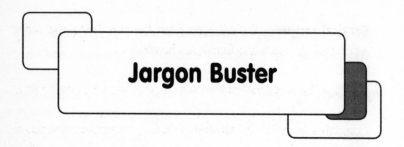

Jargon Buster

Listed below are the meanings of terms that may be used in connection with fertility and conception.

Adrenal glands – there are two adrenal glands in the human body, situated on top of the kidneys They produce several important hormones and deal directly with the body's mental and physical stress.

Amenorrhoea – the absence of menstruation.

Amino acids – organic acids that form the building blocks of proteins.

Anovulation – the absence of ovulation.

Artificial insemination – the insertion of seminal fluid into the vagina, cervix or uterus by means other than sexual intercourse.

Assisted conception – any procedure where doctors assist with the conception process.

Assisted reproductive technologies – procedures that involve processing human eggs and sperm (or both) to help an infertile couple conceive a child.

Basal body temperature – the temperature of the body at rest taken immediately on waking before any activity.

Cervical mucus – the secretion from the cells lining the cervix, which change due to the female sex hormones.

Cervix – the lower part of the uterus that projects into the vagina.

Cognitive behavioural therapy (CBT) – a treatment that targets negative thought and behaviour patterns.

Embryo – the initial stages of development of the unborn baby from the fertilised egg to around eight weeks after conception.

Endometriosis – a condition in which tissue similar to that normally lining the uterus is found outside of the uterus, usually on the ovaries, Fallopian tubes, and other pelvic structures.

Fertile phase – the days of the menstrual cycle when sexual intercourse may result in pregnancy.

Follicle-stimulating hormone (FSH) – a hormone that stimulates immature eggs within the follicles to start growing.

Glycaemic index (GI) – a ranking of foods according to the effects they have on blood sugar levels.

Hormones – chemicals produced by glands to carry messages to various organs in the body.

Human chorionic gonadotrophin (hCG) – one of the main hormones unique to pregnancy. The developing embryo produces it at its earliest stage. Its main action is to maintain the corpus luteum and the secretion of oestrogen and progesterone until the placenta has developed enough to take over.

Insulin – this is a hormone that helps your body use glucose. Glucose is a type of sugar that gives you energy. Insulin keeps the levels of glucose in your body steady. Insulin also helps glucose to be carried in your blood, so that the glucose can get into your cells. People who have diabetes do not have enough insulin or do not react to insulin strongly enough. This means they can get too much glucose in their blood.

***In vitro* fertilisation (IVF)** – assisted conception takes place in a glass dish outside of the body.

Laparoscopy – A surgical procedure in which a slender, light-transmitting instrument, the laparoscope, is used to view the pelvic organs or perform surgery.

Luteal phase – the post-ovulatory phase of the menstrual cycle characterised by the growth and development of the corpus luteum.

Multiple pregnancy – a pregnancy in which there are two or more fetuses.

Ovarian hyperstimulation syndrome – a condition caused by overstimulation of the ovaries that may cause painful swelling of the ovaries and fluid in the abdomen and lungs.

Oestrogen – the female reproductive hormone produced mainly by the ovaries.

Ovary – one of a pair of female sex glands which produce ova nad the female sex hormones oestrogen and progesterone.

Placebo – an inactive substance given to study participants to compare its effects with those of a treatment, or so they can benefit from believing they have received a treatment and will therefore feel better.

Polycystic ovary syndrome (PCOS) – polycystic ovary syndrome is a problem that affects a woman's ovaries. Eggs stored in the ovaries grow into small lumps called cysts. This can stop the eggs leaving the ovary and can cause infertility. Women with PCOS also have an imbalance in their hormones.

Primary infertility – the inability to conceive a child after one year of unprotected intercourse in couples who have no children.

Progesterone – a hormone produced mainly by the corpus luteum in the ovary following ovulation.

Secondary infertility – being unable to conceive when you've already given birth to at least one baby.

Sexually transmitted disease – any infection that is transmitted by intercourse or sexual contact.

Testicular biopsy – a procedure to obtain a sample of tissue from the testicles.

Testosterone – a hormone produced by the testes, and the ovaries. It is the main male sex hormone.

Ultrasound – a test in which sound waves are used to examine internal structures.

Uterus – or the womb in which the fertilised ovum implants and grows during the duration of pregnancy. If the ovum does not implant the uterine lining (endometrium) is shed during menstruation.

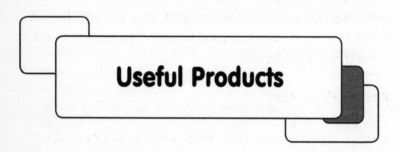

Useful Products

Below is a list of products and suppliers of products that may help fertility. The author doesn't endorse or recommend any particular products and this list is by no means exhaustive.

Australian Bush Flower Essences

Similar to Bach Flower Remedies but, as the name implies, derived from Australian plants and containing a mixture of plant essences to deal with particular conditions. She Oak promotes female balance and is recommended for the inability to conceive for non-physical reasons.
Website: www.ausflowers.com.au

Bach Flower Remedies

A system of 38 flower remedies that corrects emotional imbalances: negative emotions are replaced with positive ones.
Website: www.bachflower.com

DuoFertility Advanced Fertility Monitor

This sensor, worn like a patch, takes up to 20,000 body clock readings a day and transfers the data to give a clear visual readout of your fertile days for a full week ahead.
Website: www.duofertility.com

FertilAid

US-based company offering all natural formula preconception vitamins and antioxidant supplementation support. Also sells FertiliTea and FertileCM to improve the quality and quantity of your cervical mucus.
Website: www.fertilaid.com

FertilCount for Men

This male fertility test is a rapid diagnostic test of sperm concentration in semen. Sperm count is widely recognised as the major indicator of the fertility in men.
Website: www.babystart.co.uk

G. Baldwin & Co

Herbalist founded in London in 1844. Offers a wide range of herbal supplements, tinctures, oils and tea bags.
Website: www.baldwins.co.uk

Greenbrands Cleaning Cupboard

Offers 100 per cent natural 'green', non-toxic cleaning products without the chemicals for the home.
Email: lois@greenbrands.co.uk
Website: www.greenbrands.co.uk

Natural by Nature Oils

Aromatherapy oils produced without chemicals or parabens.
Website: www.naturalbynature.co.uk

Herbs for Healing

A Gloucester-based company with an online shop selling medicinal plants and dried herbs, as well as herbal bath and skin products and the equipment and ingredients to make your own. The website contains useful information about the medicinal properties of herbs and herbal recipes.

Website: www.herbsforhealing.net

Nelsons Homeopathic Pharmacy

Online shop selling homeopathic remedies including Nelsons' products, Duchy Herbals and Bach Flower Remedies, as well as made-to-order remedies. There is a London clinic and a shop in Dublin.

Website: www.nelsonshomeopathy.com

Opti-Omega 3 (TG) 500 mg

Supplement containing omega-3 in a highly concentrated and purified form.

Website: www.healthspan.co.uk

Ovulation & Fertility Thermometers

There is a variety of thermometers on the market to try, such as the ovulation and fertility thermometer.

Websites: www.mumstuff.co.uk
www.fertilityuk.org.

Proxeed Plus

A supplement to optimise sperm health with ingredients proven to play an important role in sperm performance including amino acids, zinc and folic acid, vitamin B12 and an antioxidant complex for protecting sperm from free-radical damage.

Website: www.valuemed.co.uk

Preparing for Pregnancy CD Set

This CD set by Glenn Harrold MBSCH Dip C. H. and Janey Lee Grace uses acclaimed hypnosis techniques to guide you into a deep state of

mental and physical relaxation – with an inspirational reading to help anyone endeavouring to become pregnant.
Website: www.hypnosisaudio.com

Pre-seed Personal Lubricant
Considered the only 'safe' vaginal lubricant for couples to use whilst trying to conceive as it does not harm sperm or interfere with fertilisation.
Website: www.preseed.co.uk

Rio Peruvian Maca 500 mg capsules
Rio Peruvian Maca is a highly nutritious root that comes from the mountains of Peru. High in vitamins, minerals and amino acids, it is a useful supplement for boosting male and female libido.
Website: www.mumstuff.co.uk

Sanatogen Pregnancy
This range from Sanatogen offers vitamin and mineral supplements for mothers- and fathers-to-be.
Website: www.sanatogenpregnancy.co.uk

The Billings Ovulation Method
A means of natural fertility that does not require any counting, temperature taking, drugs or devices and is taught over the Internet. The system records your data and displays an updated copy of your chart.
Website: www.woomb.org

The Diet Plate
A plate specially designed to help you control portion sizes and eat correctly balanced meals, thus aiding weight control.
Website: www.thedietplate.com

Tisserand Aromatherapy

This company offers a wide range of good quality essential oils.
Telephone: 01273 325 666
Website: www.tisserand.com

Viridian Fertility For Women
(Pro-Conception) Vegetarian Capsules

Formula specifically designed to provide essential and appropriate nutrients to support a woman of reproductive age.
Website: www.goodnessdirect.co.uk

Zestica Fertility Lubricant

Specifically formulated for couples trying to conceive, this lubricant uses hyaluronic acid (HA), a naturally occurring element of vaginal mucosa which plays an important role in sperm motility and sperm selection.
Website: www.accessdiagnostics.co.uk

Helpful Books

Barnes, Belinda, *Beautiful Babies, Fabulous Families, Wonderful World* (Foresight Association for the Promotion of Conceptual Care, 2010) – this book by the founder of the Foresight Association is based mainly on nutrition but also on other areas like hidden infections and electromagnetic pollution.

Glenville, Marilyn, *Natural Solutions to Infertility: How to Increase Your Chances of Conceiving and Preventing Miscarriage* (Piatkus, 2001) – contains a simple four-month pre-conception plan covering important tests, supplements and dietary advice that will increase your chances of conceiving.

Kaye, Dr Philippa, *The Fertility Handbook* (Sheldon Press, 2010) – written by a doctor with a special interest in obstetrics and gynaecology, this is a comprehensive and balanced guide to the causes, tests and treatments for infertility.

Weschler, Toni, *Taking Charge of Your Fertility: The Definitive Guide to Natural Birth Control, Pregnancy Achievement and Reproductive Health* (Harper Perennial, 1995) – this book looks at understanding fertility awareness, maximises your chances of conception before you see a doctor and provides you with information to understand your menstrual cycle and cervical secretions.

West, Zita, *Fertility & Conception: A Complete Guide to Getting Pregnant* (Dorling Kindersley, 2003) – Zita West, a midwife, nutritionist and acupuncturist, is one of the best known fertility experts in the country. This is a very useful book that leads you through the options and choices available for natural conception, fertility treatment and IVF featuring complementary and conventional therapies.

West, Zita, *Zita West's Guide to Getting Pregnant: The Complete Programme from the Renowned Fertility Expert* (Thorsens, 2005) – a useful book explaining the mind–body link with fertility, full of emotional support, medical information and advice on complementary remedies, diet and lifestyle.

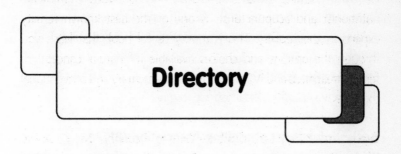

Directory

Below is a list of contacts offering information, support and products for increasing fertility.

The British Acupuncture Council (BAcC)
The leading regulatory body for the practice of traditional acupuncture in the UK.
Address: 63 Jeddo Road, London, W12 9HQ
Telephone: 02087 350 400
Website: www.acupuncture.org.uk

The British Association of Dermatologists
Willan House, 4 Fitzroy Square, London, W1T 5HQ
Telephone: 02073 830 266
Email: admin@bad.org.uk

The British Complementary Medicine Association (BCMA)
Supports therapists of any recognised therapy, providing they adhere to the code of ethics and discipline and meet training requirements. It holds a register of qualified and insured therapists.
Address: PO Box 5122, Bournemouth, BH8 0WG
Telephone: 0845 345 5977
Website: www.bcma.co.uk

British Fertility Society

The British Fertility Society is a national multidisciplinary organisation representing professionals in the field of reproductive medicine.

Address: 22 Apex Court, Woodlands, Bradley Stoke, BS32 4JT
Telephone: 01454 642 217
Email: bfs@bioscientifica.com
Website: www.britishfertilitysociety.org.uk

British Infertility Counselling Association (BICA)

BICA is the only professional association for infertility counsellors and counselling in the UK. It seeks to promote the highest standards of counselling for those with fertility problems before, during and after treatment, and for those who choose not to undergo any kind of medical intervention.

Address: 111 Harley Street, London, WIG 6AW
Telephone: 01372 451 626
Email: info@bica.net
Website: www.bica.net

British Nutrition Foundation (BNF)

The BNF was developed over 40 years ago and imparts information on the effects of food and nutrition on health through science and education.

Address: High Holborn House, 52–54 High Holborn, London, WC1V 6RQ
Telephone: 02074 046 504
Email: postbox@nutrition.org.uk
Website: www.nutrition.org.uk

Cancer Research UK

A charity dedicated to cancer research. They offer a service to cancer patients and their families, health professionals and the general public.

Telephone: 02072 420 200

Website: www.cancerresearchuk.org

Childlessness Overcome Through Surrogacy UK (COTS)

A voluntary surrogacy organisation founded in 1988 which helps couples through surrogacy.

Address: Moss Bank, Manse Road, Lairg, IV27 4EL

Telephone & Fax: 0844 414 0181 (local rate call) or 01549 402 777

Website: www.surrogacy.org.uk

Daisy Network

The Daisy Network Premature Menopause Support Group is a registered charity for women who have experienced a premature menopause.

Address: PO Box 183, Rossendale, BB4 6WZ

Email: daisy@daisynetwork.org.uk

Website: www.daisynetwork.org.uk

Donor Conception Network

A self-help network offering support and advice from parents whose own children were conceived by donor insemination, for those contemplating or undergoing treatment.

Address: PO Box 7471, Nottingham, NG3 6ZR

Telephone: 02082 454 369

Email: enquiries@dcnetwork.org

Website: www.dcnetwork.org

Endometriosis UK

This charity provides information and support to women suffering from the condition endometriosis.

Address: 50 Westminster Palace Gardens, Artillery Row, London, SW1P 1RR

Telephone: 02072 222 781

Helpline: 0808 808 2227

Website: www.endometriosis-uk.org

Fertility Friends

An online charity providing free support services to couples using assisted conception, or considering adoption, surrogacy or living without children.

Website: www.fertilityfriends.co.uk

Fertility UK

The National Fertility Awareness and Natural Family Planning Service to the UK.

This service provides comprehensive and objective information to the general public and health professionals on all aspects of fertility awareness and natural family planning for women and couples. You can also search the website for a local NHS fertility awareness practitioner.

Address: Bury Knowle Health Centre, 207 London Road, Headington, Oxford, OX3 9JA

Email: admin@fertilityuk.org

Website: www.fertilityuk.org

Foresight: The Association for the Promotion of Preconceptual Care

With over 30 years experience, Foresight has developed a thoroughly researched and successful programme to restore fertility. The association promotes the importance of optimising health to obtain a natural conception.

Address: 178 Hawthorn Road, Bognor Regis, West Sussex. PO21 2UY

Telephone: 01243 868 001

Website: www.foresight-preconception.org.uk

The Human Fertilisation and Embryology Authority (HFEA)

The HFEA is a government organisation that regulates and inspects all UK clinics that provide fertility treatment, including the storage of eggs, sperm or embryos.

Address: 21 Bloomsbury St, London, WC1B 3HF

Telephone: 02072 918 200

Email: admin@hfea.gov.uk

Website: www.hfea.gov.uk

Infertility Network UK

The UK's leading infertility support network, offering face-to-face and telephone information and support to anyone affected by fertility problems at national and regional level. By writing to I. N. UK (with a SAE to the address below) members can request a medical opinion on their condition or treatment received. Various factsheets and other sources of information are available on the website.

Address: Charter House, 43 St Leonards Road, Bexhill on Sea, East Sussex, TN40 1JA

Telephone: 0800 008 7464

Advice Line: 08701 188 088

Website: www.infertilitynetworkuk.com

www.ivf-infertility.co.uk

This website is designed by infertility specialists mainly for couples who are experiencing fertility problems and think they may need medical help.

IVF World

An online service that rates infertility clinics based on real life stories. Patients rate their experiences in different categories. You can find a clinic or just friends through the service.

Website: www.ivfworld.com

Dr Marilyn Glenville PhD:
The Natural Health Website for Women

Dr Marilyn Glenville is a registered member of the Nutrition Society, author and psychologist and recognised as a leading UK nutritionist, specialising in women's health. She is a patron of the Daisy Network, a charity for premature menopause.

Address: 14 St Johns Road, Tunbridge Wells, TN4 9NP

Telephone: 08705 329 244

Website: www.marilynglenville.com

The Medicines and Healthcare Products Regulatory Agency (MHRA)

A government agency responsible for ensuring that medicines and medical devices work and are safe.

151 Buckingham Palace Road, Victoria, London, SW1W 9SZ

Telephone: 02030 806 000

Email: info@mhra.gsi.gov.uk

Website: www.mhra.gov.uk

The Miscarriage Association

The Miscarriage Association provides support and information to all those who have lost a baby.

Address: c/o Clayton Hospital, Northgate, Wakefield, West Yorkshire WF1 3JS

Helpline: 01924 200795 (Mon–Fri, 9 a.m.–4 p.m.)

Website: www.miscarriageassociation.org.uk

National Institute of Medical Herbalists (NIMH)

The UK's leading professional body representing herbal practitioners that promotes the benefits, efficacy and safe use of herbal medicine.

Elm House, 54 Mary Arches Street, Exeter, EX4 3BA

Telephone : 01392 426 022

Email : info@nimh.org.uk

Website: www.nimh.org.uk

NHS Direct

NHS website offering an online initial assessment where you can check your symptoms and get health advice. The website links to NHS Choices, which has a healthy-living section with advice on dealing with infertility and includes specialist advice on treatments and tests. You can also find out about support in your area. They also link to fertility tests online and ovulation predictor calculators.

Website: www.nhsdirect.nhs.uk

Royal College of Obstetricians and Gynaecologists

This professional body encourages the promotion and study of obstetrics and gynaecology.

Address: 27 Sussex Place, Regent's Park, London, NW1 4RG

Telephone: 02077 726 200

Website: www.rcog.org.uk

Smokefree
An NHS clinic offering advice and support to help quit smoking.
NHS Smoking Helpline: 0800 022 4332
Website: www.smokefree.nhs.uk

TAMBA
The Twins and Multiple Births Association is a charity set up by parents of twins, triplets and higher multiples and interested professionals. They help parents and professionals meet the challenges that multiple birth families face.
Address: 2 The Willows, Gardner Road, Guildford, Surrey, GU1 4PG
Telephone: 01483 304 442
Website: www.tamba.org.uk

Women's Health Concern Ltd
A charity offering online information on women's health issues including sexually transmitted diseases and infertility. Also offers email and telephone advice.
Address: Women's Health Concern Ltd, 4–6 Eton Place, Marlow, Buckinghamshire, SL7 2QA
Telephone: 01628 478 473
Website: www.womens-health-concern.org

Zita West Clinic
Midwife, nutritionist and acupuncturist Zita West is a renowned fertility expert. The Zita West Clinic is the UK's most successful integrated reproductive health clinic.
Address: 37 Manchester Street, London, W1U 7LJ
Clinic Telephone: 02072 240 017
Telephone: 0870 166 8899
Website: www.zitawest.com